Cardiological Dilemmas

Roger Blackwood
MA, BM, BCh, FRCP

and

Bev Daily
MB, BS

BEACONSFIELD PUBLISHERS LTD
Beaconsfield, Bucks, England

First published 1995

British Library Cataloguing in Publication Data
Blackwood, Roger
    Cardiological Dilemmas
    I. Title II. Daily, Bev
    616.12

ISBN 0–906584–40–X

Phototypeset by Gem Graphics, Trenance, Mawgan Porth, Cornwall in 10 on 12 point Times.
Printed in Great Britain at the Alden Press Ltd., Oxford.

Acknowledgements

We would like to record our warm thanks to our colleagues Dr Kim Fox, Dr Peter Havelock Dr Patrick Kerrigan and Dr John Lloyd Parry. Each of them read the original manuscript in detail and made numerous helpful and constructive suggestions, which we were glad to be able to take into account when preparing the final version. On occasions we found that one would write 'Rubbish' and another would write 'Excellent' against the same answer, indicating that we are all human and that, on this particular occasion, we may have achieved a consensus.

In seeking to learn what we do not know
we are greatly hindered by what we do know.

Claude Barnard (1843–1878)

Preface

Our first book together, *What Shall I Do? Questions and Answers in Cardiology*, consisted of a series of questions posed by a GP and answered by a cardiologist. The questions were based on common, everyday problems that might be encountered by a GP in his or her surgery, for which no answer could easily be found in a standard textbook. Questions such as 'How long after a heart attack would it be safe for my patient to go and watch his team play in the Cup Final at Wembley?' or 'A hypertensive patient wants to learn the trumpet. Should he?'

No sooner had the cardiologist snorted 'That's stupid. Nobody asks daft questions like that!' when into his outpatients walked a hypertensive man asking whether it was safe to play the trumpet!

This book is written in the same vein. The questions range from the mundane to the slightly esoteric, taking account of some of the recent advances in cardiology. Questions such as . . . 'Which patients might be suitable for a heart transplant?', 'Is it safe to start ACE inhibitors at home?', 'Should we anticoagulate all our fibrillating patients?' . . . to the more worldly . . . 'Who should shovel the snow off the path, husband or wife?', or 'Should a doctor pay as much for his new stethoscope as he does for a new golf club?'

It is hoped that this little book, like its predecessor, will pose some of the questions you would like to ask and give some of the answers you would like to hear.

It must be emphasised that this is not a textbook, but a book of opinions, with which some, or many, will disagree. But the opinions are honestly held – even if, from time to time, the tongue slips slightly into the cheek.

R.B., B.D.

Contents

Contents

Contents

Aspects of Ischaemia

1. **A man comes into the surgery and says, 'Doctor. I've been looking at a medical book and I read about something called "Silent Myocardial Ischaemia". Now I'm afraid I might have it.' The doctor asks 'What symptoms do you have?'. The patient replies 'None. That's what I'm worried about!' Please explain this paradox.**

There is nothing worse than feeling perfectly well and being turned into a patient, by your doctor, for something you never knew you had. This is sometimes unavoidable – with hypertension and significant hyperlipidaemia, for example. In these circumstances, silent ischaemia is a particular cardiological variety of eye-wash that can well be done without by patient and doctor alike.

A few years ago it was noticed that some people, on 24-hour ECG monitoring, demonstrated ischaemic changes in the ST segment for which there were no corresponding ischaemic symptoms; no angina, whence 'silent ischaemia'. It was thought that as a result the heart would become damaged in some way and, more importantly, in a way that was avoidable. It was suggested that such people should be treated in a similar fashion to those who actually experienced angina. There is no evidence that such an approach makes any difference to the well-being or longevity of the persons involved. For everybody's sake it is better to leave them as they are, i.e. as people who feel perfectly well, rather than as patients with the ever-present anticipation of dropping down dead. With one exception . . .

Prognosis from a myocardial infarction is directly related to the size of the infarct. The infarcting process may continue without the patient having any symptoms. If, in the 24 hours following an infarct, the ST depression lasts longer than an hour, then the patient suddenly enters a much higher risk group. He requires an angiogram very quickly and may need an urgent angioplasty or coronary artery bypass graft.

In most other cases, once additional hazards such as hypertension, severe hyperlipidaemia and smoking have been excluded, silent ischaemia is probably best ignored, not least because nobody knows what it actually is. 'Where ignorance is bliss, 'tis folly to be wise.'

2. **A doctor is spending a holiday with his friends in the Scottish High-lands. It is winter and they are snowed in. The host, a man of 60, has a myocardial infarct and, although the pain is not severe, goes into LVF. Help will be some time coming. The doctor has his bag with him and gives his friend frusemide 20 mgm i/v. His friend remains breathless and has creps + in both lungs. Another 20 mgm is given. No improvement. Another 20 mgm is given. The friend is still in acute failure. What does the doctor do now?**

The same as what he should have done earlier – give some diamorphine, say 5 mgm i/v and 5 mgm i/m, ideally with 12.5 mgm i/v of prochlorperazine if he has it. The question says that the man is not in a lot of pain, but that is not the entire point. Diamorphine does reduce pain, but it also allays anxiety and, most importantly from a cardiovascular, hydrodynamic point of view, it drops the pulmonary artery pressure, reduces the after-load and thus reduces the strain on the heart.

I would give another 20 mgm of frusemide, but unless the patient has been on diuretics already, little further improvement is to be expected after 60 to 80 mgm. If the patient has been on diuretics for failure prior to the MI, a dose as big as 250 mgm, given slowly, might be required.

This man must be got into hospital as soon as possible. Clot-busting aside, he is going to need something like dopamine to raise his pressure, get his renal flow going and save his life.

If all else fails, two Boy's Own manoeuvres would be to cuff his legs and prevent venous return and, even more spectacular, bleed him of a couple of hundred mls of blood. Both measures would slightly reduce the load on the heart. Remember, too, that the man must be kept in the correct position, i.e. sitting up rather than lying down.

3. **A toolmaker of 47 years develops troublesome angina which is difficult to control with medication. Whilst awaiting investigation he suffers a myocardial infarction, from which he recovers well. After the MI he has no more angina, even though he takes no therapy. Is there a reasonable explanation for this?**

The apparently paradoxical situation of being better after a heart attack than before is not that uncommon. It might be described as 'a therapeutic infarction', much in the same sense as embolisation is used in the treatment of vascular problems by some radiologists, except that in this case the happening is a natural event rather than doctor-induced.

Commonly the patient has one-vessel disease, perhaps from a congenital stricture. It may only be a minor branch, but the piece of heart muscle it supplies becomes increasingly ischaemic and complains with more and more angina. Eventually the vessel occludes completely, perhaps death occurs to only a very small part of the heart muscle, the cardiac function is not affected and the patient makes a complete recovery. There is, of course, no more angina as there is no living ischaemic tissue.

The infarcting vessel might, however, represent a particularly severe area of generalised coronary atheroma, and in all cases a coronary angiogram should be carried out to find the status of the other vessels. But not uncommonly they are found to be relatively healthy. In such cases, if proven, even the insurance companies may take a more than usually generous attitude towards the 'patient who has had a previous myocardial infarct'.

4. **A librarian of 60 is admitted to hospital with a central chest pain which she describes as 'uncomfortable but not unbearable'. The pain lasts for two hours. The pain is thought to be cardiac in origin. Both ECG and cardiac enzymes reveal no gross abnormality. A diagnosis of 'First onset angina' is made. Can you explain this diagnosis?**

This is another example of cardiological eye-wash. There always has to be a first attack of angina in someone who is going to develop the condition. More often than not it is short in onset, relatively mild and strictly related to effort. But not always. Anginal attacks can be prolonged, particularly in unstable angina, which I suspect is the case here.

The first attack of angina has no particular mystical significance, although something is made of the diagnosis by some physicians . . . 'First episode angina' and the like.

The important consideration, of course, is not to miss a myocardial infarction in which the pain may not be very severe, nor associated with sweating, nor with changes in the pulse, nor with a fall in blood pressure. If a person such as the above was seen at home then she should certainly be treated, and referred, as a myocardial infarct – a diagnosis which cannot be excluded without serial enzymes and ECGs (to be done straight away, at 24 hours and at 48 hours).

The most important thing in this case is to establish an accurate diagnosis, which 'first onset angina' is not. The patient, as soon as is reasonably thought safe, must have an exercise test. At most units this would probably be six weeks after the initial event.

A certain number of patients with prolonged, non-infarction, ischaemic attacks are bound, by the very nature of things, to receive streptokinase in those units where it is given very early on. This is the price to be paid for treating infarction with streptokinase in the vital first hour (see Question 17), before any of the infarction indicators have become positive.

5. **A coronary angiogram is described as showing coronary artery spasm. Is this spasm in any way related to the spasm shown by vessels in migraine or Raynaud's phenomenon? Is there any connection between coronary artery spasm and these other conditions? Should ergotamine preparations be withheld from a patient suffering from coronary artery spasm? How does the risk of having an infarction from coronary artery spasm compare to that which results from an atheromatous blockage?**

There is no association between coronary artery spasm and these other conditions. Raynaud's, for example, works at a microsopic level which is nothing like the gross constriction involved in coronary artery spasm. Maseri at the Hammersmith Hospital tried to show a connection, but was unable to do so. Coronary artery spasm seems to be something entirely on its own.

How do we know it exists? If suspected, a coronary angiogram is carried out and during the investigation ergonovine is injected into the catheter. The normal reaction of coronary vessels is to constrict by approximately 30%. In coronary artery spasm the vessels will constrict down to 70–80% below their normal bore, sometimes closing down almost completely, necessitating an urgent dose of vasodilator into the catheter!

There is a risk of myocardial infarction in people with coronary artery spasm, but not as great as in those whose symptoms are due purely to physical, atheromatous blockage. That having been said, coronary artery spasm invariably occurs in those parts of the coronary vessel where there is some atheroma present. There seems to be something in the atheroma which affects the relaxation factor in the endothelium of the blood vessel, the EDRF, making spasm more likely.

Although there is no relationship with migraine, ergotamine preparations should *never* be used in patients with coronary artery spasm, nor, indeed, in patients with any form of angina. The same applies to sumatriptan. It goes without saying that people with coronary artery spasm absolutely must not smoke. Neither should they be prescribed nicotine patches or nicotine chewing gum.

6. **A keen golfer with ischaemic heart disease consults his GP. He says he enjoys his game except that at the third and twelfth holes – both hilly – he gets angina and some breathlessness as he walks up the slope. He stops half way and usually recovers quite quickly before making his way to the top. To miss these two holes means that he will be excluded from all the club competitions. What should the doctor advise?**

The doctor should certainly advise that he goes on playing the game and enjoying himself. Angina is a warning sign. There is nothing wrong with exercising until it starts and then having a rest. He will do himself no harm. That is not to say that he should exercise until the pain is so bad he has to stop. That is an entirely different matter and could well end up with him having an infarct.

I would advise him to take a GTN tablet (or use a GTN spray) two or three minutes before driving off on the hilly holes. If it was very cold and he found himself getting pain on the first fairway, I would advise against continuing the round. A cold wind against him could be particularly nasty.

This is an ideal circumstance for him to treat himself to an electrically-powered trolly, or to join a club with a flatter course.

7. **What are the differences in symptoms, development and prognosis of the various forms of myocardial infarction ... anterior, inferolateral and inferior. Should the doctor advise and treat the patient according to the type of infarct?**

If I were to have a coronary I would prefer to have an inferior infarct, because that would only involve the right coronary artery and the smallest amount of heart muscle. An anterior infarct covers the largest area and causes the most amount of damage. With an anterior infarct you are more likely to have a tachycardia and go into failure. As the prognosis of an infarct depends upon its size, the smaller the better.

An inferior infarct often slows the heart down, making the infarcted area require less oxygen and extension, therefore, is less likely. An inferolateral infarct, in both geography and severity, is between the two. As far as the patient is concerned, the symptoms of all three types of infarct are the same. The classic, though not always ever-present typical ECG changes are ... Anterior infarct – Q waves, ST segment elevation and T wave inversion in leads V1 to V6. Inferior infarct – same changes in leads 2, 3 and AVF. Inferolateral infarct – same changes in leads 2, 3, AVF, V5 and V6.

All are treated in exactly the same way.

8. A factory manager of 45 mentions that on several occasions he has had a pain 'like a lump in the chest', usually when he becomes very excited, or, on one occasion, when he tried to lift a very heavy weight single-handed. You feel sure he has angina. The exercise test is negative. Would you do anything further?

The answer here, first and foremost, is that angina is a diagnosis made principally on history and not just on exercise-testing. If you think the man has got angina, that is much more important than the result of the exercise test. The exercise test may be falsely negative for a variety of reasons. The man, for example, might not have been pushed hard enough during testing. If you think that he has angina you must proceed to a thallium study (an isotope method of showing up areas of myocardial ischaemia) or – quicker, and simpler in the long term – get an angiogram done and establish the diagnosis once and for all.

It is not uncommon for people to have mainly emotional angina with little angina of effort. This apparent paradox almost certainly arises from the pathology of angina. It has been suggested that angina can arise from a fixed lesion or a dynamic lesion. Imagine for example that a man has very narrowed arteries, the likely consequence of which is that every time he exerts himself he will get ischaemia and, therefore, pain.

In some people there is a considerable element of potential spasm (see Question 5). Spasm is nearly always associated with an area of atheroma. The area of atheroma, however, might not, under ordinary circumstances be sufficient to cause angina on effort, but when the area is further narrowed by spasm caused by a sudden rush of adrenaline, resulting from excitement or argument, marked ischaemia – and chest pain – can result.

9. An airline pilot of 50 returns from a trip to the Far East. He says that during an argument on the flight deck he experienced an aching pain across the chest radiating into his jaws which lasted for twenty minutes. He did not tell anybody about it. You have him very fully investigated. A coronary angiogram shows neither blockage nor spasm. What decision would you make about his future?

If this man has a normal coronary angiogram and, presumably, has had a normal exercise test, with this history I would arrange a thallium scan. If that were also normal, I think I would have to say that he had no significant coronary artery disease and allow him to continue to fly.

The only other possible cardiac explanation for this pain is that he does have angina in the presence of normal coronary arteries, the so-called 'syndrome X'. This is a condition possibly due to small vessel disease or changes in the myocardial cells themselves. Patients with Syndrome X do not have an increased incidence of dropping dead, though they might have pain. In my opinion, even if he was thought to have Syndrome X, this would not be a reason for him to stop flying.

Chest pain, particularly during periods of stress, must be one of the greatest problems for GPs to deal with, the ultimate 'is it or isn't it?' We have often discussed what might be called 'Chest pain of adulthood', a condition comparable to 'Abdominal pain of childhood'.

The latter is fairly well demarcated; the pain around the umbilicus, the type of child – tending to be thin rather than fat, female rather than male, obsessive and nervous rather than extrovert – and usually occurs around the age of 8 to 12 years. There is a complete absence of physical findings.

Chest pain of adulthood is multifactorial. I would not include in this diagnosis patients with gastro-oesophageal reflux because they can present their own particular difficulties, not least because the pain of oesophageal spasm can be relieved by nitrates and the fact that eating can bring on angina.

This is a different group entirely. The pain is usually felt in a specific part of the chest, often the left side – the left mammary pain. Often there is a localised tenderness in a Tietze-like distribution over the sternocostal joints or over the thoracic spine. The pain is sometimes postural, sometimes made worse by deep breathing.

But in the vast majority of cases the clincher is that the pain is either present all the time or 'Worse when I sit down. It goes off when I get up and do something.' There is absolutely no relationship between the pain and effort, although there may be between the pain and emotion, in which case it should be fully investigated.

As already stated, angina is a diagnosis made on the history. The association between effort and pain is the *sine qua non* of angina. Any pain experienced between the xiphisternum and the eyebrows, including arms, hands and fingers, brought on by effort, I would regard as angina until proved otherwise.

Patients with chest pain of adulthood are usually fit young men, often under strain. Strong reassurance may work, but they often have to undergo a fierce supervised exercise test, without dropping dead, before they are really convinced that they are OK. All that being said, I think I would prefer to travel on a plane not flown by a man subject to chest pain, whatever the case.

10. **Ischaemic heart disease is said to be more common in the Type A personality than in the 'laid back' type of individual. Is it likely that medical attempts to reduce the stress in Type A's is likely to increase their prognosis from a cardiovascular point of view?**

Type A personalities are the descendants of the village warriors, quick to action, easily 'fired up', calling on their large, available stores of catecholamines. They are not, unlike the descendants of the pastoral people, the shepherds, happy to wait at the back of the queue, suffer fools gladly, be tolerant of poor service, other road users or of other people's opinions.

There is more and more evidence that the Type A personalities do have more coronaries than the Type B's. This ischaemic heart disease in Type A's is, I feel, intrinsic to the way they are made, and altering them with psychotherapy, tranquillisers and the rest isn't going to make much, if any, difference. They should be aware of their A-type nature and the risk that it carries and be taught to take more care of themselves, particularly with regard to such things as smoking. Try to divert some of their Type A energy towards personal health promotion.

11. **A man of 48 has an acute chest pain in the middle of the night, which his GP diagnoses as 'Acute indigestion'. The pain eventually goes but two days later he feels ill and rather breathless. He is hospitalised. The chest pain had, indeed, been an MI and further investigation shows that he has sustained considerable damage to the left ventricle. 'If only you'd have been given streptokinase the other night the damage would not have been nearly so bad', says the young hospital doctor. Is he correct?**

This question holds a number of medico-legal implications, not only regarding the long-term effects of missing a myocardial infarction, but also the damage that might be caused by withholding streptokinase or similar medication.

If the patient died the same night negligence might be considered, as rapid treatment with 'clot-busting therapy' (see Question 18) considerably improves the prognosis at the early stages. If the patient has survived for two more days the treatment would not be given in any case.

There is no hard evidence that streptokinase and the like have much effect on the size and extension of the infarct, though it seems reasonable to assume that they might be beneficial in this context if given early enough in the infarct.

There is, however, one important factor that can definitely lead to the infarct extending more than it otherwise would have done, and that is any kind of work performed by the myocardium either from mobilisation of, or effort by, the patient.

Even in these enlightened days the post-infarction patient is kept resting for a day or two. The fact that this man was misdiagnosed meant that no advice was given to him to limit his activities, and by default it could have led to him damaging himself.

A diagnosis of indigestion, with no previous history, made on a patient with chest pain, severe enough to call out a doctor in the middle of the night, could be construed as cavalier, at least, if not frankly negligent.

Sometimes, unfortunately, in these circumstances the patient will say 'I'm sure it's indigestion, Doctor'. But that should not be allowed to confuse the issue.

Finally, I would hope that my junior hospital staff would think carefully before saying things that might be injudicious.

12. **A man of 68 presents to his GP with early heart failure of recent onset. The GP can find no cause and starts him on a diuretic. Almost immediately the man feels much better. A week later the man drops down dead with a myocardial infarction. Is such failure preceding an infarct a common occurrence? Above what age (if any) would you consider it *not* necessary for a patient in early, unexplained failure to be referred for a hospital opinion and investigation?**

Myocardial infarction very, very rarely presents as failure first. There may be preceding pain, a reduction in exercise capacity or even a vague malaise, but not overt failure. After all, the *sine qua non* of a myocardial infarct is so often its devastating unexpectedness! If only we did have more warning.

The GP here has been very unlucky, as it could appear to the family that he has missed something. I would say, however, that if the patient was young when he presented with failure, in his early forties for example, I would take some investigative action straight away . . . which brings me to the second half of the question.

When or whether to investigate? To investigate somebody is pointless unless you are going to act upon the result of that investigation. There is nothing likely to be found at the investigation of a 95-year-old hemiplegic slowly drifting into failure that is going to change your treatment. A previously well 75-year-old rapidly going into failure may, on investigation, reveal a tightening aortic valve, the replacement of which could give another ten years or more of good life.

When a patient presents with failure you should exclude obvious non-cardiac causes such as anaemia, hypertension or thyroid dysfunction. The age is not as important as the general fitness of the patient, the speed of onset of failure, and the probability of a treatable cause.

In an ideal world, the majority of new heart failures are worth referring not least because of the hospital availability of echocardiography. Modern treatment of heart failure with diuretics and ACE inhibitors is so successful, and can be so life-enhancing, that the opportunity should not be missed.

Generally speaking, although diuretics are more effective in early and mild failure and should be the first drug tried, such are the beneficial effects of ACE inhibitors that they are considered by most cardiologists to be very under-used in practice. If hospital referral results in a wider use of ACE inhibitors, so much the better.

13. A woman of 54 comes to her GP in an aggrieved state. She has had chest pain for a year. The pain has not been particularly related to effort or emotion, has been mainly on the left side of the chest and has, on occasion, been associated with chest wall tenderness. In view of her concern she has been referred to a cardiologist. Her husband of 59, with a rather similar chest pain, had been referred to the cardiologist a year previously. The lady was upset because, although the cardiologist had ordered an exercise test for her husband, he had not thought it necessary to do so for her. Was her upset medically justified?

This is going to sound a very sexist answer! Not doing a treadmill test was medically justified . . . but it would take a brave man to refuse her.

It is becoming apparent that chest pain in women is notoriously difficult to assess. Men are much easier. If you were to take a large group of men and women, of varying ages, all with what we would define as classical or typical angina, and did angiograms on them all, 7% of the men would be found to have normal coronary arteries. Quite a lot, you might suppose, in a condition so clinically clear to diagnose. But in the case of the ladies – 40%! That is, 40% of women with classic symptoms of angina do not have recognisable ischaemic heart disease on angiography.

Furthermore, of female patients who have symptoms reasonably suggestive of angina, 60% have normal angiograms. If you take a group of women who, like the one in the question, have chest pain not suggestive of heart disease, they are no more likely to have an abnormal angiogram than women of the same age who have no symptoms at all.

It can be argued, therefore, that doing an exercise test on a female patient with non-anginal chest pain is not justified on the symptom of pain alone. But I would, not only for reassurance purposes, but also in case she dropped down dead in the next two or three years.

Remember. The largest number of fatal heart attacks occur in people who have relatively minor ischaemic heart disease. They are more common, percentage-wise of course, in those with severe atheroma. But there are millions of people with relatively minor IHD and thousands and thousands of them have fatal coronaries, as much as a result of bad luck as anything. I suspect that a high proportion of fatal MIs in a GP's practice are suffered by people, particularly in a younger age group, whom nobody suspected of having anything wrong with them.

There is one group of younger women that I do get fussed about, apart from those with terrible family histories. They are the ones who take oral contraceptives and are heavy smokers. There are quite a lot of them about. And they *can* drop down dead.

14. A man of 62 has had occasional, fairly mild, easily controlled angina for four years. It has bothered him very little. He has not had a coronary angiogram, but an exercise test two years previously did not suggest a severe, imminently life-threatening degree of IHD. Recently, although the angina has been no worse, he has found that he gets rather dizzy if he walks up a slope or exerts himself more than a little. Should this be a cause for concern?

Very much so. This man almost certainly has main stem disease. This would be shown up on a carefully regulated exercise test, when his BP would begin to fall after only a little effort. This is exactly what is happening to him in real life. Effort equals drop in blood pressure equals dizziness.

His angina might have not got any worse. I have, however, never seen dizziness as a symptom of ischaemic heart disease when there was no angina at all. In aortic stenosis, on the other hand, dizziness alone might present.

This man needs an urgent exercise test and will almost certainly go on to angiography and CABG (angioplasty is not indicated in left main stem disease). Diagnosed correctly, you might, literally, give him many more years of life.

15. A somewhat reclusive man of 60 has a chest pain lasting three hours. ECG shows an inferior infarct. He refuses to go into hospital. In the cottage in which he lives his bedroom is upstairs, the lavatory is downstairs. He works in a factory doing a fairly heavy job. What plan of mobilisation would you give him?

I would give him a clearly laid out set of instructions. The bed must be brought downstairs . . . not by him! He must live on one level.

1) The first week he spends on bed rest, just getting up to go to the loo.
2) The second week he can get up and toddle about downstairs, but not go outside.
3) The third week he can go out and walk around his garden, assuming that it is not a hundred acres and as long as the weather is not cold or very windy.
4) The fourth week the house and garden are unrestricted, and he should walk half a mile a day.
5) The fifth week . . . house, garden, and walk a mile a day.
6) The sixth week . . . house, garden and walk two miles a day.

He should attend outpatients at the end of 6 weeks, by which time he should be getting back to normal. When he goes back to work depends upon the nature of the job. If it is very heavy he might need a few more weeks off. The aim, however, is to get the patient back to the job that he was doing before the infarct . . . as far as the law (on driving or flying, for example) and all other circumstances allow. Apart from anything else this has a very strong beneficial psychological effect.

At 6 weeks an exercise test should be carried out, and if that is significantly positive angiography should be arranged. This is particularly important before a patient goes back to a heavy occupation.

Of course, one has to say that this advice is flavour of the month – it is the regime recommended at present. Previous regimes have varied from prolonged total bed rest to very rapid mobilisation . . . all of us know people who have taken no notice of their doctors and gone back to work the day after an infarct, with no apparent harm. But we do know that early exercise can extend an infarct, thus worsening the prognosis, and the above would seem a reasonable compromise.

One further point. In a case like this, the help given by a kindly neighbour, who will keep an eye on the man, perhaps bringing him one hot meal a day, is more valuable than gold.

6. **A bank manager of 50 has been seen at the local cardiology clinic for an episode of chest pain. You are told it is thought that he had a sub-endocardial infarct. Should he be advised any differently from someone who has had an ECG proven infarct?**

This is old-fashioned cardiology in the sense that infarcts used to be classified as 'full-thickness' or 'sub-endocardial'. Originally it was thought that the patient had damaged either the whole thickness of the heart wall or just the inner third.

Now we differentiate between 'Q wave infarcts' or 'non-Q wave infarcts' . . . the latter being a description of anything that is not a 'Q wave infarct'.

The mortality figures from the two types of infarct, at the time of the original attack, are quite different – Q wave about 10%, non-Q wave about 3%. However, over the next 12 months the non-Q wave mortality catches up until both stand at about 15%. The diagnosis of non-Q wave infarction is made on the symptoms (the same as any other infarct), the enzyme changes and any minor ECG changes that there might be.

It is very important that sub-endocardial infarcts are followed up carefully with exercise tests and so on, and that there is a very low threshold for angiography. Hopefully, in these circumstances, something may be done early enough to prevent the non-Q wave infarct entering the area of worsening cardiac risk.

As far as the management was concerned, I would treat this man in the same way as I would treat any other person with an infarct. I would give him as much rest as possible, and would not allow him back to work for at least 6 weeks after the event. At 6 weeks I would also carry out an exercise test.

Clot-Busting, Clot Prevention

17. A recently-retired man of 63 has a fairly acute chest pain strongly suggestive of a myocardial infarction, but will not go into hospital unless his disabled wife is also hospitalised. She refuses admission and a 'stand-off' situation develops. Would you advise the GP to give the man some 'clot-busting' therapy at home? If such a therapy were to be embarked upon, what precautions should be taken?

Let us first consider the advantages of 'clot-busting' therapy. Various studies have suggested that:

1) If the treatment is given within 1 hour of the infarct the mortality can be reduced by 50%.
2) If the treatment is given 6 hours after the infarct the mortality is reduced by up to 25%.
3) If the treatment is given 12 hours after the infarct the mortality is reduced by 12%.

Thereafter the improvement in prognosis no longer justifies the treatment.

There are three major problems in giving 'clot-busting' therapy at home:

1) Not infrequently, reperfusion of the ischaemic cardiac muscle can cause arrhythmias, notably ventricular fibrillation. Unless, therefore, the doctor is in a position to defibrillate at home, an unnecessary death may result.
2) The treatment may produce significant hypotension, and this could be very difficult to deal with in an ordinary bedroom situation.
3) Usually streptokinase is the drug given, TPA (tissue plasminogen activator) being prohibitively expensive for the average GP to carry as an emergency drug. Streptokinase has to be given as a monitored perfusion over 1½ hours, something that is very difficult to manage at home.

No, I would not give this man anything but the diamorphine that he required for the pain and a half an aspirin a day – the first to be chewed as soon as I had made the diagnosis – and try to ensure that he had as much rest as possible. Otherwise, if something goes badly wrong it may well be perceived that the treatment has killed him.

8. **A dentist who has a strong family history of heart disease, but has no other particular markers himself, becomes very anxious at the possibility of having a myocardial infarction. His cousin has just had streptokinase therapy for an MI. He asks how such cases are dealt with in your local hospital. What do you tell him? What if he were 75 years old? What if he had mitral stenosis and was on long-term warfarin?**

I would describe to him the following scenario . . .

An ambulance turns up at A & E. Inside is a man with a severe pain across the chest. Hopefully the admitting medical officer is already waiting. He takes a quick history ascertaining, as far as possible, that it is a typical infarct. He asks whether there is a history of bleeding tendency, recent surgery, history of recent CVA or CVA with residual disability, recent indigestion, current peptic ulceration, severe liver disease, oesophageal varices or diabetic retinopathy. All these are contraindications to streptokinase, the last-mentioned because of the risk of sudden blindness in the affected eye(s). At the same time a line is being set up and an ECG performed.

Satisfied that it is most likely an MI, he gives the patient a strong analgesic (preferably diamorphine in a dose dependent on whether or not he had been given any prior to hospitalisation), an aspirin to chew (if he has not already had one) and examines him. He will hopefully exclude the more obvious pneumothorax, dissecting aneurysm and abdominal crisis. He will take particular note of the diastolic blood pressure. If it is 110 or above he will not give streptokinase (it could cause a brain haemorrhage). At this point, no contraindications being present, he will consider giving streptokinase.

This is where different units may vary. Some will demand changes suggestive of infarction on the ECG before they go ahead. However, in view of the critical time element (the 50% increase in survival rate given by streptokinase in the first hour following the onset of chest pain), some units will start such therapy on history alone, e.g. a crushing chest pain that has been present for 30 minutes, with or without ECG changes.

It must be ascertained whether or not streptokinase has been given to the patient in the previous twelve months. If it has, it will have provoked antibodies that will make its re-use ineffective. There is also an outside possibility of anaphylaxis. If streptokinase has been given in the previous 12 months TPA must be used.

If the decision to use streptokinase is made then hydrocortisone 100 mgm i/v is given, followed by 1½ million units of streptokinase i/v over the next 1½ hours. The patient must be carefully monitored for reperfusion arrhythmias (see Question 17).

If the man was 75? Contrary to some of our earlier thoughts on the matter it now seems that the elderly particularly benefit from streptokinase, as do those patients with the larger infarcts. Simply, the older you are and the iller you look, the more you need streptokinase. Any and everybody except the groups mentioned above should have streptokinase or TPA after an infarct.

If the patient was on warfarin I would not consider that to be a contra-indication for the use of streptokinase.

19. A doctor in his morning surgery sees two men. The first is 55 years old with no evidence of cardiac disease at all. He does, however, have chronic atrial fibrillation. The other, 73 years old, also fibrillating, has a known cardiomyopathy. The doctor is concerned that one, or both, should be on warfarin. Are there any general rules on deciding who should, and who should not, be anticoagulated?

Before the general discussion, a thought about these two cases. I think that both should see a cardiologist and have an echo. The first in order to make absolutely sure there is no visible, structural abnormality. If there were no abnormality I do not think he needs anticoagulating. The older man needs careful assessment and a decision to give him anticoagulants will most likely be made.

The problem of atrial fibrillation and anticoagulation is a very difficult one indeed. In the last few years, there have been five major trials on this particular issue and a quick summary of all of them is that, on average, the incidence of emboli on placebo is about 5% per annum, whereas the incidence on warfarin is about 2% per annum.

Trials included all types of patients with atrial fibrillation whatever the cause, although only a few had lone fibrillation. (Lone fibrillation means that people have been fully examined for evidence of any other heart disease and none has been found.) In all the trials there was quite a wide variation of anticoagulation, from an INR of 1.4 right up to 4.2.

The first thing to point out about these trials is that the annual bleed rate from situations where people are being anticoagulated is 1.7%. These major bleeds, in a sense, should be added on to the warfarin percentage before comparing it with the placebo percentage. This brings up the difference between placebo and warfarin to 5% against 3.7%. This immediately reduces the absolute justification for anticoagulation and makes it not, perhaps, quite as impressive as at first sight. A number of other problems presented in these trials.

Firstly, there were very few patients under the age of 50, and it is known that in this age group the risk is very low for any form of embolus. It is therefore reasonable to state that under the age of 50, it would not be justifiable to put fibrillating patients on anticoagulation without some other pressing reason, such as a prosthetic valve. In only two of the trials were patients with lone fibrillation considered, and in this group there were no emboli noted at all.

Perhaps one of the biggest problems with anticoagulation is the feasibility of circumstance. There were a large number of withdrawals from the trials, and if we were to anticoagulate all patients who have atrial fibrillation over the age of 70 we would be anticoagulating 10% of that part of the population! Locally I have calculated that this would require us to have another eighteen anticoagulant clinics a week to cope with the load. Since this is completely impractical, one really must look for some form of risk stratification and decide who would be the best people to have warfarin.

The trials suggest strongly that if there is any structural abnormality associated with the fibrillation (increased left atrial size, increased left ventricular size, poor function etc.), then the risk of having an embolus is significantly increased. This also applies to hypertension and other heart diseases. Warfarin must therefore be considered where atrial fibrillation is associated with known cardiological disorder. We do not yet know whether aspirin has any part to play in such cases.

It is reasonable from this to say that all new cases of fibrillation should be seen by the cardiologist and given an echocardiogram. Certainly those over 60 with structural heart disease should be considered strong candidates for warfarin. It takes about 8 hours for a clot to form in the left atrium once atrial fibrillation occurs, so a person who has paroxysmal atrial fibrillation with very short attacks is in much less danger than one who has longer attacks.

I have not mentioned rheumatic heart disease in this answer. It goes without saying that all such patients, if fibrillating, must be anticoagulated without delay.

20. Due to a shortage of staff, the local hospital asks GPs to manage most of their own patients on anticoagulants. There seem considerable differences of opinion on what should be done as the INRs go up and down. Is there any simple protocol that can be used in the adjustment of warfarin dosage?

There are no simple tables that can guide a doctor to the appropriate anticoagulant dosage. It has to be a matter of common sense and experience – that is why anti-coagulant clinics are so useful, dealing as they do with the same problems all the time. Most doctors alter the degree of the patient's anticoagulation, to a certain extent, according to the problem in hand:

Prosthetic heart valves	INR between 2.5 and 4.0
Pulmonary emboli	INR between 2.5 and 3.5
Systolic emboli ⎱ DVT ⎰	INR between 2.0 and 3.0

It is usual to start the anticoagulation with warfarin 10 mgm, 10 mgm, 5 mgm on three consecutive days, whilst the patient is also receiving heparin. Exceptions to this would include hepatic disease and – especially in cardiology – the concomitant use of amiodarone. Here 5 mgm, 5 mgm, 2 mgm would be safer. In those cases where the patient does not need urgent anticoagulation, for example the decision to start anticoagulants for a long-standing mitral disease, the warfarin can be started, at home, with an initial dose of 5 mgm a day.

It takes 48 hours to register an INR change with warfarin, and initially daily measurements of INR may be needed after the third day. The regular daily dose of warfarin can vary from 1mgm to 15 mgm or more. It should always be taken at the same time of day. Sudden changes in INR most commonly occur with infections, especially gastrointestinal, and when other drugs have been given (fully covered in interaction tables in BNF). Amiodarone has already been mentioned in this context, and if started the warfarin dose should immediately be halved.

Adjustments of warfarin dosage are usually made in the order of 1 to 2 mgm. If the INR goes over 5, stop the warfarin for 48 hours and restart on half the previous dose, and then readjust.

Generally, the giving of vitamin K is not a good idea as it often more than reverses the warfarin for a variable amount of time. This could result in a patient's prosthetic valve becoming clotted up. If the patient is bleeding with an INR of 5+, fresh frozen plasma i/v in hospital is the best treatment.

Medications Old and New

1. Mr Smith returns to the surgery every couple of months or so for some 'fresh heart pills'. He has rarely used more than one or two. Is there a place for the continued use of sub-lingual glycerine trinitrate, or are the modern alternatives superior? Why not always use sprays?

Why not indeed? The answer is purely economic. GTN tablets are dirt cheap. Furthermore, if the patient mislays them or runs out, he can always go to the chemist and buy some more without a prescription, costing himself less than the average prescription . . . and costing the NHS nothing at all. A bottle of GTN, however, should be thrown away eight weeks after being opened, whereas the trinitrate sprays are not only convenient but also have a long shelf and pocket life. Nor are the sprays particularly expensive at about a fiver.

The only other disadvantage of some trinitrate sprays is that they can cause soreness under the tongue. If I had angina I would certainly prefer a spray (or two) and would expect my doctor to prescribe accordingly, even if he was a fund-holder!

2. Why mononitrate *and* dinitrate?

Both, of course, can be used to relieve the pain of ischaemic heart disease. When it comes down to it, there is little to choose clinically between mononitrates and dinitrates. Theoretically the dinitrates, which were the first on the scene, are said to get rapidly chewed up by the liver. This does not apply to mononitrates. In practice, however, there is very little difference, and it is best to be guided by what the patient prefers and what the doctor is used to giving . . . and which is the cheaper.

Certainly the serum levels with mononitrates remain high through day and night. The problem with this is that it can lead to tachyphylaxis (the ability of the body to become adjusted to a medication, so that it is no longer affected by it).

For the person who has to take a nitrate on a very regular basis, it is probably easier to give a medication that is formulated to be taken once a day. There are several mononitrates in this category, and attempts are made in their absorption profile to keep tachyphylaxis down to a minimum.

19

23. You are confronted by a new patient asking for a fresh supply of his blood pressure pills. He has taken them for years, he tells you, and feels very well. His blood pressure is well controlled. The tablets are methyldopa. How would you react? What if they were propanolol?

Firstly, there is no justification whatsoever for changing his treatment. The main reason for changing a hypotensive, and indeed your main consideration when you first put a person on such medication, is the amount and severity of side effects involved. If the patient's blood pressure is well controlled and he is complaining of no side effects, you would be barmy to change his medication, however 'old-fashioned' you construed it to be. You must of course be sure that there really are no side effects. Problems like impotence might not have been admitted to, and a direct question may be necessary.

Secondly, there is no difference between any of the tablets used to treat blood pressure when it comes to their effect on life expectancy.

Thirdly, of all the factors that most increase the risk and prognosis in hypertension, probably the most important is left ventricular hypertrophy. Of all the drugs that are used for treating hypertension, methyldopa is one of the most efficient, over a period of time, at reducing such hypertrophy, second only, in this context, to ACE inhibitors.

As far as the propanolol is concerned, the same argument applies – happy on the pill, hypertension well controlled, don't change.

It is worth mentioning that there are now said to be four generations of beta-blockers. The first includes propanalol and oxprenolol, the second includes drugs like atenolol with a few less side effects, the third includes bisoprolol and finally, the fourth and most recent, drugs such as celiprolol, which have not only less side effects but also have a vasodilating characteristic not present in the other beta-blockers. The payoff in changing, however, may not be as good as it seems. By the time you have reached celiprolol you may find a lot less side effects but you might not find much beta-blocking either.

You do not change from one beta-blocker to another, everything else being equal, unless the side effects are bad.

4. A retired headmistress of 80 years has taken atenolol 50 mgm daily for mild hypertension and 'heavy beating of the heart' since the age of 66. Her BP is now 140/90. She no longer has any 'heavy beating'. Would you leave her on beta-blockers into her eighties? If so, for how long?

This is another situation for not changing a winning team. If the lady feels perfectly happy on a beta-blocker, at the age of 80, leave things as they are. If you take her off the beta-blocker she will, almost certainly, have a bad period of time where the increased circulating adrenaline will knock her sideways with sweats, heart pounding etc. This could last for several months. Some of these elderly patients cannot live in any comfort without beta-blockers. If this lady had other conditions coming on which can be made worse by beta-blockers, such as intermittent claudication or severe Raynauds, you might think about it. Not otherwise. And you would of course re-evaluate the whole situation if she showed any sign of heart failure.

The elderly do benefit from the treatment of their hypertension, which is – usually – systolic. The best medication for treating systolic hypertension in the elderly is a beta-blocker.

5. Thiazide diuretics provide a safe, smooth treatment for many elderly hypertensives. Is their effect on lipid levels sufficiently deleterious to make their prescription generally inadvisable?

The short answer is 'No'. The change in the lipid levels will amount to 5–10% in the wrong direction, and in this group of patients the increase in risk will be very small.

A modestly raised cholesterol, by itself, in the elderly patient is not a great risk factor. If the patient, however, smokes forty cigarettes a day, has a poorly controlled blood pressure and a bad family history, one should not make things worse by increasing the lipids, and here one might look for a different medication . . . but, there again, most of these individuals are not likely to have reached 'elderly'!

6. What indications are there for using verapamil? Apart from beta-blockers are there any other drugs with which it should not be used? Does it have any particular advantage in the treatment of hypertension?

Verapamil is a very good drug, but being rather old-fashioned tends not to be very trendy and is sometimes overlooked.

First of all it is an effective hypotensive, as good as any other. Its disadvantage is that it tends to make people feel tired and, particularly, it does cause constipation. Secondly it is very good for angina, especially where the beta-blockers cannot be used – in an asthmatic, for example. It is the strongest of the calcium antagonists in this context. Thirdly it is very effective in controlling supraventricular arrhythmias.

It is therefore a useful drug covering a broad area. Its advantage in the treatment of hypertension is that whereas many drugs do have disturbing side effects, the only really significant side effect of verapamil is constipation and that can usually be overcome with a few prunes for breakfast. Nifedipine is more commonly used in hypertension, however, because it can be used with beta-blockers. Similarly diltiazem is generally preferred in angina because it, too, can be used with beta-blockers. If verapamil is used with a beta-blocker you may get a straight line on the ECG, i.e. a cardiac arrest. Do not use verapamil with a beta-blocker. There is no other drug with which it cannot be used.

Care has to be taken in heart failure, where it might make things worse. Verapamil is often the drug of choice in supraventricular tachycardia.

27. **A doctor looks in his bag and finds that the lignocaine he carries for cardiological emergencies is out of date. Is it worth replacing for future use? Should he be carrying something else instead?**

I do not think there is any justification for carrying lignocaine in a GP context unless a sophisticated monitoring system is also available. Lignocaine is used in the treatment of ventricular arrhythmias in a hospital context. There is no evidence that giving lignocaine i/m has any preventive role with regard to ventricular fibrillation.

If I was a GP and was faced with a patient who had an MI and a tachycardia I would send for the ambulance and, whilst waiting, give him an aspirin to chew and some intravenous diamorphine. The diamorphine tends to lower the pressure in the pulmonary artery and slow down the heart rate. I would, most likely, also give some intravenous prochlorperazine. Ten years from now I might also be giving a safe clot-buster at this time (there are more than forty such substances currently being developed).

It must be remembered, however, that 30% of the population of the UK live more than half an hour away from a hospital, some much more. There also has to be a wait for the ambulance. Many GPs working in these circumstances have both a portable ECG and/or a defibrillator. In these particular circumstances lignocaine might be appropriate.

8. In spite of evidence to the contrary, some old people do seem to tolerate quite large doses of digoxin. Are some old people more sensitive to digitalis intoxication than others? Are there situations that might make such intoxication occur in an unexpected fashion, and what should the GP look out for? How often should an elderly patient with digoxin on a repeat prescription card have his digoxin level checked?

I don't see much digoxin overdosage these days, because most doctors are aware that as patients get older their daily dose of digoxin should be reduced. For the average, elderly patient the little blue tablet of 62.5 micrograms digoxin is quite sufficient. I don't use a loading dose. Some people can be given higher doses, indeed can benefit from them; but as a general rule, if the advised dose of digoxin for a particular age was not working, I would be looking towards another drug.

Older patients with decreased renal function do not clear digoxin as efficiently as younger patients. Many are on diuretics, and the effect of the serum potassium on digoxin levels becomes an added factor.

There is no doubt that the most important sign of digoxin toxicity is nausea. If I see a patient on digoxin with nausea, in whom there is no other obvious cause, I stop the digoxin straight away, even before getting any blood tests back. The classical sign of digoxin overdosage is bigeminal rhythm, where the patient has a normal beat followed by a ventricular ectopic.

My feeling is that if an elderly patient is not responding to 62.5 micrograms of digoxin I wouldn't increase it further. Up until ten years ago I used to see the occasional patient who was being given as much as 750 micrograms digoxin a day, with no particular benefit, but not, surprisingly, getting much in the way of side effects either.

I do not think measuring digoxin levels in the absence of symptoms is of much value. Much more important, for the patients on repeat prescriptions of digoxin, is for them to let you know if they have any feelings of nausea. They should then be checked straight away for bigeminal rhythm, etc.

29. Germany is not known for being backward-looking in the way it deals with problems. Is it correct that German doctors prescribe far more cardiac glycosides and far more nitrates than we do? Might they be right to do so?

The Germans use more digoxin than we do, and very much more in the way of nitrates. Curiously, I think, as far as the the digoxin side of things is concerned, that it has become a habit amongst some doctors to prescribe the drug for people who feel a bit weary and unwell and who could just be in borderline heart failure, a prescribing habit that does not exist in this country. A high proportion of patients in heart failure are prescribed digoxin, much as they were here before the advent of modern diuretics. Such diuretics are of course available and prescribed in Germany, but German doctors go on using the digoxin as well. Digoxin, similarly, is used very frequently in France for the treatment of heart failure.

Germans generally choose nitrates as their first line treatment in angina far more than we do, because they really believe that they work very well, whereas we feel we should start our patients on beta-blockers. In the end, of course, a large number of patients in both countries will end up on triple therapy – nitrate, beta-blocker and calcium antagonist.

30. A man arrives in the surgery having worked for fifteen years in France. You find that he is hypertensive. He says that his boss, in France, had the same problem and was prescribed alpha-blockers, having been told by his doctor that they were 'much safer than beta-blockers'. What advice would you give him?

This answer to this question rests on to two matters. What are the side effects of alpha-blockers and beta-blockers? And how effective are they?

With beta-blockers there is the risk of some bronchospasm, peripheral vasoconstriction, leaden legs, weariness and dreariness and breathlessness of unknown cause. There might be some interaction with other drugs that the person is taking, there might be some effect on the lipids, there might be an effect on the person's heart failure, and so on.

Alpha-blockers have much less in the way of side effects – first dose hypotension, perhaps, or the occasional rash. So far so good. The main snag is that the effectiveness of the alpha-blockers is nothing like that of the beta-blockers. They are less effective as hypotensive agents and have virtually no effect on angina or arrhythmia. It's a 'You pays your money and you takes your choice' situation. I rarely use alpha-blockers except, occasionally, doxazosin as a second-line treatment for hypertension.

Perhaps the reason the French manager preferred the alpha-blocker is that it is free of one side effect which is often laid at the door of its beta brother. Impotence! On the contrary, alpha-blockers, being vasodilators, might even have the opposite effect.

1. A man of 54 has an obvious heart attack in Marks and Spencers. Whilst awaiting the ambulance he is attended by a GP who has come in to buy a new shirt. The GP does not have his bag with him but he does have – indeed, habitually carries – some soluble aspirin in his pocket. He offers one to the man to chew. The man declines, saying that he has a duodenal ulcer from which he has fairly recently had a haemorrhage. Should the doctor push him? Apart from this acute situation, are there any circumstances in which you do not give aspirin, in the long term, after an MI?

All GPs should, at all times, carry soluble aspirin … not the micro-encapsulated form, designed for long-term use without irritating the stomach, because it is not absorbed quickly enough. Aspirin taken within the first half an hour following an MI confers as much prognostic advantage as (and, of course, in addition to) that provided by streptokinase, with all its expense and technical expertise involved.

Aspirin should be chewed so that it can be rapidly absorbed 'all the way down'.

In the case described, however, if the man had had an ulcer bleed in the previous few weeks I would not give the aspirin. It only takes a very small dose to start an ulcer bleeding again, and an MI complicated by a bleeding ulcer would not be a happy situation. In almost any other circumstance I would give the one dose of aspirin. If he just suffered from indigestion I would certainly go ahead.

In the long term I would not give aspirin to people on warfarin, to people who had had recent surgery, or to those who had blood dyscrasia or diabetic, proliferative retinopathy.

If, post-MI, I had to give ranitidine, or omeprazole or the like, to enable the person to take aspirin, I wouldn't bother with the aspirin. It would mean two medications instead of one, and I think that the increased 'invalidisation' of the patient would not be justified by the improvement in prognosis.

Diagnostic Aids

32. A patient has an appointment to go to the hospital for an echo-cardiogram. He says he has already had an ECG and doesn't want to go again. What's different about this test, he wants to know, and will it tell the specialist anything new?

An echocardiogram is basically a radar picture of the heart which shows up both abnormalities of structure and function. The ECG gives little information on structure, except for suggestions of factors like ventricular hypertrophy, but it does give information on conduction abnormalities and ischaemia, which the echo does not. The two are complementary, and echoes will be done more and more as part of any cardiological assessment. The test is completely painless and free of any harmful radiation.

The ultrasound waves (2.25–6 mHz) are emitted from, and picked up by, a transducer placed over the 4th left intercostal space. The waves bounce off the various surfaces of the heart and produce a moving picture of the chambers and vessels.

The test is non-invasive, cheap and repeatable. It is therefore of particular use in keeping an eye on a potentially changing situation such as that encountered with a gradually closing aortic stenosis. A stethoscope can detect aortic stenosis, but an echocardiogram with Doppler (see below) can show you just how much blood is flowing through the valve. Across the aortic valve, for example, a gradient of 25 mmHg would mean mild disease, 50 mmHg moderate, and 75 mmHg, or over, severe disease that most likely requires surgery.

Amongst the structural abnormalities that can be detected are congenital abnormalities. The viewing of a small VSD, for example, may obviate the need for catheterisation.

In the adult, chamber size is most important and is covered in the questions on cardiomyopathy (Question 81) and on hypertension with cardiac enlargement (Question 37). From the GP's point of view, echocardiography can be a quick (fifteen minutes) way of determining whether or not a patient's breathlessness is due to heart failure. Abnormalities of valves can be visualised, as can such conditions as pericardial effusion – the best method of investigating this condition.

It is not a particularly useful test in the context of investigating childhood murmurs, most of which are innocent, and requires a degree of expertise that is rarely found outside of teaching hospitals or centres of cardiological excellence.

Functional changes, such as those presented by ventricular contraction, are particularly important in the assessment, and prognosis, of cardiomyopathy. The advent of Doppler echocardiography, in which flow rates are transformed into coloured signals, has proved very useful in the detection of such conditions as mitral incompetence and in the ongoing assessment of aortic stenosis.

Sometimes there can be problems with getting a good picture in patients such as the very obese, or in those with chronic obstructive airways disease. Unfortunately – as opposed to ECGs which involve some competence, of course – echocardiograms are best carried out by technicians who have considerable experience, ideally of some years and, much like the craftsmanship produced by the skilled cabinet maker, the information obtained is highly dependent on the skill of the operator.

33. A local Rotary Club collects a handsome sum of money for the local health centre. They wish the money to be spent on 'Something to do with the heart'. Half the practice want a defibrillator, the other half a diagnosing electrocardiograph. The practice is eight minutes from the nearest ambulance station and has its own, standard, electrocardiograph. Which option would you suggest? If neither, how would you spend the money?

I would not spend the money on a defibrillator. I doubt that the average practice would have an indication to use it more than once a year, and then it would, quite likely, not be to hand for the doctor confronted by the emergency. By and large, defibrillators, except in a hospital setting, cannot sit and wait for cases to be brought to them. They have to be taken to cases. The ideal transport medium for defibrillators is the ambulance service . . . and the paramedics that come with them are far more used to the equipment than the average GP.

Of the two major pieces of equipment, I would choose the diagnosing electrocardiograph, bearing in mind that this machine has to be viewed very critically. For safety reasons these cardiographs are very sensitive to any abnormality and tend to overdiagnose considerably. They can, however, usefully draw the attention of the doctor to a particular abnormality without him or her having to agree with the diagnosis. In cases of doubt the ECG can always be faxed through to the local cardiologist.

In truth, owning a standard ECG machine and being relatively close to the ambulance station, I would prefer something entirely different. I would spend the money on several home blood pressure machines and a 24-hour ambulatory ECG monitor, or an event monitor . . . or both, funds being available (see Question 65). The information I could gain from the use of these devices – and they would be in use much of the time – would not only be beneficial to my patients but also cut down on the number of hospital referrals.

34. A GP trainer is going through the notes of the patients seen by his trainee. They are clear, concise and relatively full. Amongst the notes reviewed are several cases of heart failure, both chronic and acute. There is plenty of mention of basal crepitations, breathlessness and oedema but none of JVP, raised or otherwise. When questioned, the trainee says that he never seems to remember to look. Does it really matter? How important a physical sign is the JVP or is its assessment, rather like routine percussion of the chest wall in every case of cough, a thing more of Dr Finlay's era? Should we now be looking for different things?

The JVP is one of the most difficult physical signs to evaluate. Many textbooks suggest that it is a piece of cake, you just do this and do that and then read it off as a pulsation monitor in the neck. Easy. In reality, in most cases, it is absolutely useless. It only rises in chronic heart failure and, then, only when that heart failure is quite severe. There will be plenty of other signs to look at and to listen to before the JVP is raised. The assessment of the wave form, in my opinion, is of minimal value and I quite agree that, as a physical sign, it belongs to a bygone era.

Although basal crepitations and ankle oedema are the best known and most dramatic signs of heart failure, they are both relatively late signs. A patient can be in sufficient heart failure to be breathless on minimal effort and not demonstrate either.

The earliest physical sign, apart from the symptom of breathlessness, that can suggest heart failure is a sinus tachycardia. If you see an afebrile patient who is a bit puffed with no apparent cause, and who has a sinus tachycardia of 100, the chances are that he or she is in early heart failure. If you see a breathless patient with a pulse rate of 60 the chances are that heart failure is not the likely diagnosis . . . as long as the patient isn't on beta-blockers!

These days we look for failure much earlier, as the treatments with diuretics, ACE inhibitors and so on can be so effective. Once patients have basal crepitations they have severe heart failure and are probably very breathless. If they have a raised JVP they have probably had failure for years. The same applies to peripheral oedema. These signs have become so much part of the medical catechism because our forebears, unable to do much for the heart failure in their patients, had little more to do than take gloomy notice of its remorseless progression.

With modern, rapid-acting, safe diuretics you have a very handy tool for detecting early failure. If you see somebody who is a bit breathless and demonstrates no physical signs, improvement after taking a diuretic pill almost certainly confirms heart failure. This is diastolic heart failure. Sometimes the patient may have a wheeze which is not resolving with salbutamol or the like and which magically disappears with a diuretic. The synonym of LVF is, after all, 'cardiac asthma', and one tends to forget that it can truly present as a wheeze. Similarly, older patients with a chronic cough who have had several lots of antibiotics can get dramatically better on a diuretic, demonstrating that the cough is a manifestation of mild cardiac failure.

35. The GP's car is stolen from the golf club car park. Everything has to be replaced. A man of average cardiological ability, should he spend (a) less, (b) more, or (c) the same on his new stethoscope compared to his new number 3 wood?

This is a highly academic question. Firstly it depends upon whether the GP described as 'of average cardiological ability' is also of average golfing ability. If he habitually plays off an equivalent handicap of 40, it is probably no more worthwhile his acquiring an expensive new number 3 wood than it is spending £120 on a stethoscope. Something more ordinary would suffice, as indeed would an ordinary, inexpensive stethoscope suffice for most of the cardiological problems faced by the auscultating GP.

Secondly – and somewhat more profound – there has been a change not only in the practice of medicine but also in the conditions it seeks to alleviate, and the stethoscope has now acquired a less esoteric role than it had previously. To be dying of heart disease sixty years ago more than likely meant that it was from rheumatic heart disease, which was much more common than it is now. It provided doctors with all kinds of rasps, rumbles and rattles to diagnose and prognose. There were few Hollywood films of the era which did not have a doctor, usually in Vienna, listening to the heart of the young heroine and declaring gravely, 'You have exactly fourteen weeks to live, my dear.'

Ischaemic heart disease, the grim reaper of today, provides very few clues down the stethoscope. The doctor still has to listen – intently – to what the patient is saying, because it is the nature of the symptoms which he or she describes that is of the utmost importance. Even the ubiquitous electrocardiograph, decorating most doctors' surgeries, is generally considered of little use in diagnosing anything but sub-catastrophic ischaemia and has been universally succeeded by the stress test.

It is certainly necessary to hear the important sounds of cardiovascular medicine – basal crepitations, arrhythmias and the more thunderous murmurs such as aortic stenosis – but you do not need the Rolex equivalent of a stethoscope for that. Even the most ardent cardiologist would not put his life savings on a diagnosis of mitral stenosis from a presystolic rumble at the apex when he had an echo machine in the next room.

Apart from the enthusiasts, and more power to their elbows, who might want to listen further and enjoy all the snap, crackle and pops picked up by their hi-fi instruments, the average GP would be better advised to have several inexpensive stethoscopes spread about the place so that he has always got one to hand, and does not have to press his ear directly to the chest in a manner which might lead to some distress at his particular medical defence organisation.

Hypertension

36. A keen amateur pilot of 43 years tells his GP that he has got to go to another doctor for his routine flying medical. He says he is concerned, because at a recent works medical his BP was measured at 170/100. Is his concern justified?

In any circumstance like this, the most important thing you can do is to establish, as far as possible, at what level the blood pressure is running for the majority of the time. We are all aware of 'white coat hypertension' and realise that many people can dramatically put up their blood pressure when faced with a medical examination.

The blood pressure in the case above may be a falsely high reading. There are two ways in which you can determine whether it is or not. You can use a 24-hour monitoring blood pressure device. I'm not very keen on this approach, as nobody really knows what constitutes a 'normal' variation in the day. Would you say, for example, that a person was suffering from hypertension if their blood pressure was only raised above normal for three hours in the twenty-four?

The better way to do it, I believe, is to give the patient their own automatic blood pressure machine, send them home with it for a fortnight and tell them to take three or four readings a day, at different times, so that a large representative range of recordings can be obtained. In this way I think that you can get a much better idea of what is going on. You must check the machine against a mercury manometer when you first give it to the patient, and check it again when it is returned. You ignore those occasional extraordinary readings that can be thrown up by the machine.

Returning to the man above. He probably hasn't got too much to be worried about even if his BP is found to be persistently running at 170/100. He will, however, almost certainly have to take some form of hypotensive medication and be shown to be stabilised on it.

The Civil Aviation Authority has its own list of examining doctors who are most experienced in this area. They are given guidelines of acceptable maximum blood pressure at various ages. Up to 39, 145/90, 40 to 49, 155/95, 50+ 160/100. It will depend upon the discretion of the examining doctor, however, whether they are considered safe.

There is no reason why the pilot should not control his hypotension with modern hypotensives such as the ACE inhibitors, calcium antagonists, beta-blockers and thiazide diuretics. Methyldopa is not looked upon particularly favourably, nor are the older hypotensives such as reserpine.

37. **A male company director of 47, apparently in good health, goes for an expensive private medical 'check-up'. The physical examination is essentially normal except for a BP of 160/100. The heart sounds are normal and the man admits to no undue breathlessness. The examining doctor is surprised to find that the chest X-ray reports 'some cardiac enlargement', and the ECG shows left ventricular hypertrophy. Unabashed, the doctor reassures the patient that 'Some people have big feet, some people have big hearts. It's neither here nor there.' The mildly raised BP he ascribes to the stress of the medical. Is his avuncular reaction preventing yet another case of cardiac neurosis?**

This is something you can't ignore. Here you have borderline hypertension, and that doesn't matter too much in itself, but you also have evidence of end-organ damage – enlarged heart, LVH on ECG – and that puts you in a completely different ballgame.

The chest X-ray can be confusing – you may just see a large blob. It is essential, therefore, to get an echo done and then make your decisions on treatment. A patient who has LVH is at considerably more risk from heart failure, infarct, stroke and peripheral vascular disease, than one who has not.

Approximately 5% of patients with hypertension demonstrate left ventricular hypertrophy on an ECG, whereas 30% will show the existence of true hypertrophy on an echo.

These patients must be treated vigorously. It is preferable that all patients with hypertension should have an echocardiogram. In an ideal world this would mean that all hypertensives should be referred to the cardiologist. In the real world, however, this would be totally impractical.

8. A woman of 47 has her hypertension satisfactorily controlled with a beta-blocker. She develops bronchitis. The cough does not get better and her GP finds that, for the first time, she has developed marked bronchospasm. He takes her off the beta-blocker, treats her with salbutamol and she gradually improves. She says that, until the recent illness, she felt very well on the beta-blocker and would like to go back on it again. Is the GP justified in giving it to her, or is it most likely to bring about a rapid return of the bronchospasm?

Once you have a patient who has had bronchospasm, at any time, from any cause, you will be in grave danger of killing him or her if you prescribe a beta-blocker. It is a very dangerous situation indeed – bronchospasm once, beta-blockers never again. I am quite aware that this is a severe policy, bearing in mind that a high proportion of the population have had bronchospasm at one time or another. Nevertheless, it is impossible to predict which of these people when given a beta-blocker will react in a violent, if not fatal, fashion.

It is not uncommon for people who are taking beta-blockers to develop bronchospasm when they get a chest infection. You would, of course, stop the beta-blocker immediately. Unfortunately some of these people who have never previously suffered from bronchospasm continue with it for the rest of their days, in spite of coming off the drugs.

9. As a cardiologist, which do you consider the most carefully, the diastolic or the systolic blood pressure? Might a neurologist take a different view? On your 70th birthday, many years hence, a colleague takes your blood pressure. It is 200/90. What would you do?

A raised diastolic disturbs me the most. The systolic is much more susceptible to catecholamines and the fright of the moment. If the diastolic was 100 or more all the time I would take serious note of it. With the systolic, the official level to get bothered at is 160 but I wouldn't take much notice unless it was 180 perpetually. That would be in the case of a middle-aged man.

In the elderly you are nearly always going to get systolic hypertension. This can lead to more strokes, not more heart attacks, which is why neurologists get more fussed in these circumstances than cardiologists. Reducing the systolic in such patients is said to reduce the incidence of stroke. The problem is that in spite of treatment, the blood pressure can remain stubbornly at the same high level until you fulfil that old adage,

'Shake, oh, shake the ketchup bottle, nothing comes and then a lot'll.' That is to say, you pile on the antihypertensives and, suddenly, the systolic comes crashing from 200 to about 60 and you end up with the patients having blackouts when they stand up. And this doesn't just apply to old people. This sudden drop can sometimes occur with increasing hypotensive treatment in any type of patient and take everybody by surprise.

My attitude in an elderly patient with a BP of 200/90 would be to try small doses of two or three drugs and if they didn't work, forget it. If I had a BP of 200 on my seventieth birthday I certainly wouldn't take any pills at all, not least because they might ruin what I hope would be a very active sex life. But I would certainly have a whisky.

40. Is there any hard evidence that hypnotherapy or psychotherapy or transcendental meditation have a significantly beneficial effect on hypertension?

If the operative word is 'significantly' the answer is 'No'. This kind of treatment came into vogue along with sitar music, 'Sergeant Pepper' and flower power in the late 1960s and 1970s. It was born of the idea that illnesses shouldn't really be treated with drugs at all . . . never mind the fact that many of the proponents of such ideas, and half the world with them, were spaced out on 'recreational' drugs themselves.

However much we seem to progress in medicine we, as doctors, are made to feel vaguely guilty that we are harming people, whence the popularity, for those who can afford them, of treatments that involve little more than contemplating navels, having feet massaged to cure pancreatitis, or smelling smells that will, more rapidly, mend a broken leg.

Those who did serious work on the use of meditation in treating hypertension made the fascinating discovery that it was not, as they anticipated, a decrease in circulating catecholamines that lowered the blood pressure, but a personal development of control over the vagus. It was during times of profound relaxation that one seemed to be able to do this.

The persons investigating the phenomenon, of course, tended to take the blood pressure there and then, and quite often found that it had gone down quite dramatically. Unfortunately, evidence since suggests that once the patient (or client) is out of the state of meditation, or away from the influence of the therapist, the pressure, like a roller coaster, goes rocketing back up again.

In my mind, for the person with constant, significant hypertension the judicious use of safe, well-proven hypotensive agents is, by far, the more preferable treatment. If patients wish to go off drugs and try the meditative approach, supply them with a home BP monitor and ask them to check their BP just after the milk has boiled over or their grandchild has flushed the car keys down the toilet.

1. A woman of 53 applies for life insurance. She has been under treatment for hypertension since a time, twenty-two years before, when her BP was found to be 220/110. She is heavily loaded by the insurance company. She protests, saying that she is very well – indeed, she shows no sign of left ventricular strain on ECG, no cardiac enlargement nor any retinopathy. Furthermore she says that her mother has had a high blood pressure 'all her life' and is alive and well in her eighties. Are there cases where essential hypertension really does seem to be benign?

Yes. There seem to be. But it is rather like the Grand National. Before the start we know there is going to be a winner (1993 excepted), but it isn't until the finish that we know exactly which one it is!

The problem with such benign hypertensives is that nobody can define them properly or say, except in retrospect, which ones they were likely to be. There is no doubt that some people do go through life with a higher than average blood pressure without coming to any apparent harm. But as you can't define such patients, you have to include them with the rest both from the point of view of hypotensive therapy and assessment for insurance risk.

In a case like this, an insurance company will only work in facts and figures and assess what is the life expectancy of the average woman of 53 who had a BP of 220/110 when aged 31. It has to be said that the figures on which the company bases its calculations could be twenty-five years old – because it is necessary to know the prognosis of such cases over at least that time – and might not yet represent the improved prognosis given by modern therapy. But the insurance company pays the piper and it will call the tune.

42. A rather frail lady of 64 years with a history of CVA attends a hospital clinic. She is mildly hypertensive. Every time she goes to the hospital she registers a BP in the region of 220/110. The hospital advises that she increase her hypotensive, but as soon as she sees her GP the same day it is 150/80. Should her medication be changed? What if she were a robust woman whose BP had been found similarly raised, in hospital, prior to a hernia repair?

'White coat hypertension' is now very well recognised, and almost everybody who goes to a hospital clinic will register a higher blood pressure than they will with their own GP. In this particular case, the general practitioner's reading of the lady's BP is so normal that if he were, with increased medication. to reduce her blood pressure further he might well kill her off or, at least, give her another cerebral infarction from profound hypotension.

If investigation of such a case is deemed necessary, this can be done with a 24-hour BP monitor or by giving the lady an electronic sphygmo-manometer so that she can measure her own BP at home several times a day, at different times of the day, over the next fortnight. I favour the latter. As has been said in Question 36, the problem with the 24-hour monitor, in particular, is that nobody knows what is 'normal' and nobody knows what to do if the BP is raised, say, 30% of the time. Does that represent a significant hypertension with potentially harmful effects?

As far as the fit lady with pre-operative hypertension is concerned, this can be a real pain. Countlesss people are sent away from hospital unneces-sarily, without having their operation, because of such concern. In many cases the patient is suffering from white coat hypertension which will settle down in an hour or two. If it does not, in my opinion, I would not be concerned about the blood pressure unless the diastolic was greater than 110. Even then, in the majority of cases, there is no problem. In about 25% of people with a blood pressure above that level, it may swing about a bit, either up or down, but it usually causes no harm.

Ideally the lady awaiting operation, if the blood pressure is high, should be kept in hospital for a day before surgery to make sure that things do settle to a reasonable level. If this is not possible she should be monitored (as above) at home.

43. **A GP is asked by a patient, a man of 35, to check his BP a few days before going abroad for three years. The BP is found to be 170/100. The doctor does nothing further but advises the man to have his BP checked within a month or so of arriving at his destination ... more in hope than in expectation, as he knows the man is unlikely to do this. A little over two years later he hears that the man has died of malignant hypertension. If the doctor had been more vigilant at that last consultation, might this tragedy have been avoided?**

In a case like this, the total responsibility must be placed on the patient. He must be told, in no uncertain terms, that for his own safety his BP must be monitored when he is abroad. Had he taken his doctor's advice this tragedy would have been averted.

We rarely see malignant, or accelerated, hypertension these days, as nearly everybody has their BP monitored to some degree or another. Malignant hypertension does not appear out of the blue. The patient has been cooking it up for some time and then presents at the end of the day with papilloedema, a diastolic of 140, albuminuria, incipient renal failure, perhaps hypertensive heart failure and often a clutch of neurological symptoms including confusion. Its aetiology is a neglected or unobserved, albeit fairly rapidly developing, severe hypertension.

Had the doctor checked the man's eyes and urine before his departure, it is very unlikely that he would have found any abnormality. Had the man been staying, however, and the doctor had said, quite properly, that he would check him in another month and the BP then turned out to be 210/120, suspicions would immediately have been aroused.

ACE Inhibitors

44. It is the custom of some cardiologists to admit patients to hospital when ACE inhibitor treatment is initiated, particularly for the management of heart failure. Is it reasonable to start ACE inhibitor treatment at home? What guidelines should determine the therapy and what precautions should be taken, especially with the avoidance of hypotension in mind?

There is understandable concern amongst many doctors that starting an ACE inhibitor in a patient with heart failure may be dangerous because of a precipitous drop in blood pressure. This is very rarely the case as long as one follows simple guidelines.

A sudden drop in BP will occur if the renin-angiotensin system is switched on powerfully. This would be the situation in a patient with moderate to severe heart failure on higher doses of diuretic, e.g. frusemide 120 mgm daily or bumetanide 3 mgm daily, and with a low systolic BP (<100 mm Hg). The dehydrated patient may also present a problem in this context. While the renin-angiotensin system may be switched on in lower degrees of failure it is unlikely to cause a problem.

Thus, patients with high switch-on of renin-angiotensin are those:

1) with dehydration,
2) on high dose diuretics,
3) with a low systolic BP,
4) with documented severe heart failure.

In practice, few patients are in this situation and ACE inhibitors are best started in people in early heart failure where the patient is taking, say, frusemide 40 mgm daily or bumetanide 1 mgm daily. In such cases there really is very little problem.

Practical rules:
1) Do not start the ACE inhibitor at home if the systolic BP is lower than 120 mm Hg. Send into hospital for this.
2) Either halve the dose of the diuretic or stop it altogether the day before starting the ACE inhibitor.

3) Medico-legally you have to warn people that they might feel faint when they start ACE inhibitor therapy, although it is not likely. But warn, don't terrify.

4) Start by giving the first dose at the surgery – the smallest dose of ACE inhibitor you have chosen – and observe the blood pressure. The patient will have to stay for an hour or two. Alternatively, and ideally, if you have access to day beds, use that facility. For those patients starting at night, tell them to take the pill just before they go to sleep. Do warn – particularly the elderly, who often have to get up in the night to pass water – that they might feel faint if they get up too quickly. For this reason, some doctors would prefer not to use night initiation of treatment for elderly people who live alone, lest they fall.

My own practice is to start the patient on a small dose of ACE inhibitor, such as lisinopril 2.5 mgm at home, and tell them to get on with it without any drama. I have been doing this for thirteen years without any problems, as long as I stick to these four simple rules.

45. Treated for his early heart failure with ACE inhibitors, a man of 73 develops a chronic, dry irritating cough. This does not stop until he is taken off the drugs. Although the failure is reasonably well controlled on diuretics the man says, 'In spite of the cough I felt much better on the other pills'. Would that most likely be due to his imagination?

A chronic, dry irritating cough will occur in about 20% of people taking ACE inhibitors . . . not always very badly, however, and many patients are prepared to tolerate the inconvenience because of the benefit they get from the medication. On the other hand, some people get a very bad cough and splutter every time they try to speak or get a little excited. Changing from one ACE inhibitor to another, in these circumstances, rarely, if ever, makes much difference.

People often feel much better on ACE inhibitors. This is not a placebo effect. As a result of the vasodilating effect of the ACE inhibitors the muscles are being perfused much more efficiently. The patients, as a result, feel less languid, less tired, less uncomfortable. An experience of increased well-being is achieved, as this man describes.

If the diuretic alone is not controlling the failure, and ACE inhibitors are causing an intolerable cough, an alternative is to introduce hydralazine at a dose of 50 mgm tds, perhaps associated with a small dose of nitrate. The hydralazine, as a vasodilator, confers some of the benefits of ACE inhibitor including an improved life expectancy. Digoxin, once considered an essential drug in the treatment of heart failure, is generally only useful in failure when there is either fibrillation or a tachycardia with a third heart sound and crepitations.

46. A GP sees two patients, one a woman of 81, the other a man of 56. Both have a degree of CCF. To both he gives an ACE inhibitor and a diuretic. Should the prescription be for exactly the same drugs?

If the two patients had the same degree of CCF I would, probably, give them the same ACE inhibitor and, in the end, the same diuretic.

There is an argument that, as excretion through the kidneys in the elderly is not as good as it is in the young, there is a theoretical advantage in giving an older patient an ACE inhibitor that is excreted by both the liver and the kidneys, thus preventing accumulation and sudden hypotension. In practice, however, such accumulation is not that common, and unless the patient has a raised creatinine that suggests their kidneys are not working very well, I would use the same ACE inhibitor in both. It's the old story of getting to know one drug well. All that I would ask of the ACE inhibitor is that it had a once-a-day dose, for example lisinopril.

In the case of the diuretic, I would certainly be giving frusemide to the 56-year-old man, in whom a thiazide such as bendrofluazide could cause problems such as impotence. In an old lady, however, I would probably start on bendrofluazide but, most likely, soon change to frusemide if the less powerful diuretic had not upset her in any way.

47. A cardiologist unearths his old clinical diary of ten years earlier. He finds that since then he has made a number of changes in the practice of his craft. What might they have been? What changes might he anticipate ten years hence?

The greatest changes in the way that I practice cardiology, compared to ten years ago, have been brought about by the ACE inhibitors, thrombolysis and angioplasty.

Significant changes I might anticipate in the next ten years are the development of non-invasive coronary artery imaging using MRI etc., the use of laser technology in angioplasty, and the increased use of skeletal muscle to supplement cardiac muscle to which it becomes transformed when tacked on to the heart.

I also anticipate, in the near future, a much wider use of ACE inhibitors. At the present time these drugs are considerably underused. Doctors were frightened off by the strictures that were applied when they first appeared. They are very safe drugs which can increase quality of life and actually prolong life. There are a large number of people about the place, not yet receiving them, who would gain substantial benefit from ACE inhibitors.

Investigation

48. The mother of a child of two and a half years is told that in order to establish whether or not the little boy needs heart surgery, a cardiac catheterisation has to be carried out. She is desperately worried about this, particularly with regard to the risk and the degree of distress that might be caused to the child during the procedure. How should she be advised?

Almost always the children are given a general anaesthetic for such a procedure. Apart from any distress that might be caused, the children would not stay sufficiently still for accurate pressures to be measured. The child is therefore no more likely to be upset than he would be with the pre-medication and anaesthetic that might be given for any other surgical procedure.

These investigations, however, must be done in special centres, because multiple samples of blood have to be taken in order to measure the blood gases. This can amount to a fair proportion of the child's blood volume. Careful watch has to be made to avoid hypovolaemia or dehydration. The fluid has to be replaced accurately and the whole procedure carried out at a very high standard indeed.

The risk is quoted at 0.1%. The technique used (apart from the anaesthetic and the coronary catheterisation) would be similar to that described in Question 49.

49. A woman with mild angina and a positive exercise test is advised to have a coronary angiogram. She is extremely nervous about all surgical procedures and asks you to explain what she, as the patient, will experience. She asks whether it can be done under an anaesthetic. What do you tell her?

Firstly, she may be offered the choice of going as a day case or staying the night after the angiogram. The day option is better because usually the waiting list is much shorter. As for other procedures, a mild pre-med is given, but not always, and about an hour later the patient is taken down to the catheter lab/operating theatre.

As the catheterisation is invariably done through the femoral artery, the skin in the area of the groin is infiltrated with local anaesthetic. That is, virtually, the last discomfort in the procedure that the patient will feel. A catheter is then passed into the artery. A little heparin is introduced into the catheter at this stage to prevent minor clots forming at its tip.

The catheter is passed up the artery, through the aortic valve, into the heart. The patient does not, of course, feel this. Forty cc of dye are injected via the catheter into the left ventricle. This is a left ventriculogram which takes about fifteen seconds to record on the video. This procedure is accompanied by the only other discomfort experienced by the patient. A very hot, unpleasant sensation is felt in a particular part of the body. It may be anywhere, in the head, chest, arms or even in the bottom. It lasts for only a few seconds.

This catheter is then taken out and another, with a looped end, is inserted, which hooks into the opening of the coronary artery. More dye is injected – this does not cause further flushing – and several pictures are taken of each of the arteries. This is accomplished by cameras moving around the patient at different angles.

The catheter is removed and a large thumb is placed over the femoral artery for about fifteen minutes to try and prevent arterial leakage. Following that, a soft clamp is placed over the artery for another hour. Inevitably there is a lot of seepage and it may go into the subcutaneous tissues over the whole thigh as far down as the knee. The one advantage enjoyed by the overnight stay patients is that they will be able to stay in bed until the next morning. The day-patient will be up and off encouraging more seepage and more bruising.

The technique is not done under a general anaesthetic as so little discomfort is involved.

The risk of death at a catheterisation is about .01%. The risk of arterial damage requiring surgery is about 1%. The risk of an arrhythmia – ectopics etc. – is about 5%, but there is usually no problem in dealing with the situation there and then. Occasionally there can be anginal pain if the catheter momentarily blocks an artery, but this can be resolved by moving the catheter and giving a little nitrate.

The whole procedure is very safe and lasts about half an hour.

50. A GP takes on a temporary job as a small cruise ship's doctor for 'a rest and a cheap holiday'. At sea, in the middle of nowhere, he is asked to see a passenger who is unwell with a pyrexia. The man has a dry cough but no other signs ... bar one. He has a loud murmur at the apex. He reveals that he has had a mitral valve replacement some years previously. He has no recent history of a minor surgical procedure, nor dental treatment, but he does remember pricking his thumb whilst pruning the roses a few weeks earlier. He takes warfarin 8 mgm a day. The GP has no facilities for blood culture nor for doing an INR. How should he proceed? When he returns home, what parameters should he use to decide on whether or not to do a blood culture when such a service is available?

Obviously, in this situation, the diagnosis of infective endocarditis must be uppermost in the doctor's mind. There doesn't have to be any significant history of trauma, nor of introduction of bacteria into the bloodstream, surgically or otherwise. In the majority of cases there is no such history.

Whether the heart valve replacement is metal or tissue there should not be a loud murmur. Generally the prosthetic valve will produce a soft diastolic murmur which is often so soft as not to be heard at all. A loud murmur, usually harsh, usually systolic, in such circumstanes is most significant.

Blood should be taken for a blood culture and kept in a warm place until the ship docks. A useful result may be obtained. If the pyrexia lasted for more than 24 hours the doctor should start treating blind – as we very often do in hospital long before the blood culture result comes back. The advised medication is penicillin and gentamicin given intravenously.

This is a situation where the antibiotic is more important than the risk of an upset of the anticoagulation. Again, as soon as the ship docks, an INR could be carried out with speed and necessary adjustment of the warfarin be made. Often, in the best and most controlled of circumstances, no adjustment of warfarin dosage is required.

As far as a dry-land, 'normal' protocol was concerned it is obviously impractical, and unnecessary, to do a blood culture every time anybody with a prosthesis has a pyrexia. My general rule is that if there is a fairly loud murmur I would do a blood culture after the pyrexia had niggled on for 48 hours. If there was no murmur I would wait, and make sure that the patient took his or her own temperature night and morning. If the temperature continued I would then advise a blood culture.

Heart Disease and Other Illnesses

1. **A woman of 57 has recurrent attacks of severe bronchial asthma which respond favourably to short courses of heavy-dose oral steroids (40 mgm prednisolone daily). She also suffers from ischaemic heart disease, chronic oedema and bouts of cardiac asthma. Should her diuretic dose be increased when she is on the steroids?**

Certainly. I would simply double her dose of diuretic during the course of steroids and for a week afterwards. Steroids are a potent cause of fluid retention and this effect must be countered. Remember that this applies not only in asthma but in other situations, such as temporal arteritis, where large doses of steroids are used. Where lesser doses of steroids (say 15 mgm prednisolone daily) are given in the long term, in polymyalgia rheumatica for example, then some adjustment of the diuretic will almost certainly have to be made. I would certainly keep an eye on her electrolytes and blood sugar.

2. **An insulin-dependent diabetic man of 32 is seen by his GP. He has had diabetes since he was an infant. His elder brother, also a diabetic, died of renal failure at the age of 37. The man's blood pressure is found to be 140/95. On two further occasions the BP is found to be at the same level. Should the GP take any action?**

Early-onset diabetes, however well controlled, is far from being anything but a very serious disease. Many people die young from end organ damage, particularly renal failure. It is possible, by fairly rigorous measures, to regulate the blood sugar more than we normally do, but the patient is then at greater risk from having hypoglycaemic attacks with all that entails – particularly for driving. Better-controlled diabetes means less complications, however, and it is all a matter of pros and cons.

So we do the best we can. We have the blood glucose level measured rather than just testing the urine. Insulin is adjusted for both dose and absorption. In a man like this great care should be taken to monitor the renal function.

It has been suggested that diabetics are more vulnerable to slightly raised

45

blood pressure – at levels that would be ignored in the healthy. In a case like this I would consult with my diabetologist colleagues, who I suspect would rather see a BP of 130/80 or below. This might well be achieved with a small dose of ACE inhibitor.

Note: Never forget the great cardiological pitfall with diabetes. If this man were suddenly to feel unwell and his BP was to fall, untreated, to 100/70, you would have to check his cardiac enzymes and ECG. He could well have had an MI. Silent infarcts are very common in diabetics.

53. A woman of 30 is told to stop taking oral contraceptives when she sustains a deep vein thrombosis. There is also a suggestion of a pulmonary embolus but it is not proven. She stops having periods when she is 52. At the age of 55 years she develops signs of widespread atherosclerosis and has some angina. Her doctor advises her to go on hormone replacement therapy. With her past history, would this not be absolutely contraindicated?

In my opinion, in the right form, HRT would be absolutely indicated! There is a common misunderstanding about the Pill compared to HRT. They are, in no way, the same thing. In most HRT, not only is the dose of hormones a small fraction of that used in contraception, but also it is mainly oestrogenic . . . and in those who have had a hysterectomy usually totally oestrogenic.

Oestrogens are good for the heart. They can lower the blood pressure. They are vasodilators – they do, for example, measurably increase carotid blood flow – and they protect against the laying down of atheroma. Oestrogen therapy in menopausal women reduces the incidence of myocardial infarction by 50%. In the context of oral contraceptives, oestrogens can produce clots but not, I believe, in the very much smaller amounts used in HRT. I have never seen a pulmonary embolus caused by HRT. Indeed, at the tiny dosage involved, oestrogens are quite probably mildly anticoagulant.

Progesterones are supposed to have negative effects on the heart. However, as most HRT is overwhelmingly oestrogenic, I believe that any bad progestogenic effect is more than wiped out by the beneficial effects of the oestrogens. So that almost whatever the type of HRT the woman takes, unless it is strongly progestogenic, she stands to benefit from a cardiovascular point of view. Progesterone must be part of the HRT in unhysterectomised women to prevent the risk of endometrial cancer. Many gynaecologists now adjust their HRT regimes so that only the minimum amount of progesterone required for this purpose is given.

Remember. Prior to the menopause a woman is at much less cardio-vascular risk than a man. After the menopause the risk is the same. HRT puts the woman, once more, into a situation of less risk.

54. A secretary of 54 has recently developed angina on fairly heavy exertion. If she takes care, it does not alter her quality of life. She takes thyroxine for hypothyroidism. Would you reduce her dose of thyroxine even though her TSH is within normal limits and she appears euthyroid?

No, I certainly would not. She should be maintained in a euthyroid state – otherwise her cholesterol will go up, there will be an increased deposition of atheroma and her condition will worsen more quicky than it would have done otherwise.

Her TSH should be monitored at fairly regular intervals (say every 6 months) to make sure that she is not having too much thyroxine. That would certainly make her angina worse. If her TSH was very low I would want to know her T3 reading lest she were becoming hyperthyroid. I would certainly investigate her fully and pay particular attention to her lipids. I would also consider HRT!

55. An elderly man with chronic heart failure develops an acute gastro-enteritis that is running through the family. To control his breath-lessness he takes four 'mixed' diuretic pills a day. How soon should he adjust the dose of diuretic, bearing in mind the fluid loss from his diarrhoea? Is such a reduction likely to affect his cardiac asthma?

This is a difficult situation. It would depend very much on the individual. In most cases I don't think there would be a need to change the medication very vigorously. If the man has diarrhoea he's probably not going to absorb much of the diuretic anyway, and if he's going to be dry the diuretic won't dry him out that much more.

This is not an occasion where you look at the echocardiograph or the ECG. Get back to basics. Look, instead, at the tongue. If it's dry, you really have to think about reducing the diuretics, and, particularly if the man is vomiting as well, consider the electrolyte possibilities and judge whether or not he would be better off in hospital.

On the other hand, if the man feels not too bad and the tongue is reasonable leave the diuretics alone . . . it's always difficult to know when to return to the usual dose, and delay may result in the patient going into heart failure.

If he is not severely ill but the diarrhoea continues for more than a day or two, I would certainly check the U's and E's and consider whether or not to change his medication.

56. A woman of 71 suffers from occasional cardiac asthma (paroxysmal nocturnal dyspnoea). She is a very poor sleeper at the best of times and a family upset renders her unable to sleep at all. Is there any intrinsic danger in giving her sleeping tablets for a short period, or might they aggravate her nocturnal attacks?

As long as you start at a gentle dose of a drug like temazepam I don't think patients will come to any harm. They would wake up early in any discomfort that might be coming on. I don't think they would stay asleep until they found themselves in a 'drowning' situation.

The majority of patients admitted to medical wards, many of them cardiac patients, are put on such sleeping tablets before you can say 'Night Sister', without any trouble at all. The benefits of a good night's sleep override other considerations . . . in hospital that is. Unfortunately, the poor GP has to try and wean the patients off them again once they get home – a home where there will be no attendant night nurse to give them an arm as they stumble, sleepily, to the lavatory.

57. It was always happening in the black and white movies. 'Your wife cannot survive the delivery, Mr Brown, but we may be able to save the child.' Are there any cardiological circumstances in which you would actively discourage pregnancy?

This situation does occur, thank heavens, very, very rarely. Amongst those people to whom you have to say 'No' are the cyanotic, congenital heart disease patients where there is a very high pulmonary artery pressure. Such patients are blue and breathless at rest. I do have to tell people like this that there is a much greater than 50% chance that they will die, and the baby, most likely, as well. The same applies to patients with severe hypertrophic, obstructive cardiomyopathy, although many women with lesser degrees of cardiomyopathy can deal with pregnancy and birth quite well.

There is, of course, a group with such problems as very large VSDs, or large ASDs or with severe coarctation. Such patients should be operated upon and have their defect corrected before they ever get pregnant.

Mitral stenosis is not very common amongst the indigenous population but is still found in some prospective mothers. If a prosthetic valve has been inserted, then warfarin will have been prescribed on a daily basis. Warfarin is potentially teratogenic and is contraindicated in pregnany. This problem can be overcome, however, by giving the pregnant mother twice daily heparin, 12,000 units, by sub-cutaneous injection . . . for the entire pregnancy. Even better, and more convenient for all concerned, would be to teach the lady to inject herself.

8. A male school teacher of 57 with a history of myocardial infarction some eight months previously, and from which he appears to have made a very good recovery, tells his doctor that he is going to the dentist. He will probably be having a local anaesthetic. Should the dentist be advised to take special precautions? Under what other cardiological circumstances – apart from those situations involving SBE – should the dentist modify his treatment accordingly?

In the ideal world, major surgical procedures should not be carried out on a patient, presuming a full apparent recovery, within six months of him or her having had an MI. Dental problems, however, in which a local anaesthetic is used, generally represent a very low risk. The adrenaline that the anaesthetic contains shouldn't enter the blood stream in any quantity. In the case described above the patient should be treated completely as per normal.

The advice should only be modified if the patient, following the MI, is left with severe angina, or heart failure etc. Minor problems in these circumstances could still be dealt with in the dentist's chair, but dental extraction, extensive bridge work etc. might be more safely done in hospital.

Partial Truths

59. How likely is a patient to get hypokalaemia on a loop diuretic? Hyperkalaemia on a potassium-sparing diuretic? Do we make too much fuss about potassium levels?

There is one simple rule for the 'ordinary dose' diuretic taker. Whatever the diuretic, check the patient's potassium after one month. Some people are going to be affected one way or the other and they will usually show up by that time. One small group of patients are particularly good at losing potassium, but if the potassium level is not down after a month, then the person being investigated is probably not in that group and not at particular risk. Thereafter it is not worth checking the potassium week in, week out. Once a year is probably sufficient unless the development of a symptom like fatigue might suggest it be done sooner.

At the other end of the scale is the person with very severe congestive cardiac failure who can only survive with enormous doses of diuretics. There is then, obviously, a worry about the U's and E's and creatinine. When the blood is tested it is often found that the electrolytes, sodium, potassium etc. are grossly abnormal. For this reason you may be tempted to reduce the diuretics, leaving the patient to become totally waterlogged. Better to ignore the electrolytes and let nature take its course more kindly with a very high or very low potassium. This is infinitely preferable to death by drowning from heart failure. I would only adjust the diuretic in these circumstances if the patient became nauseated from a very high urea.

If hyperkalaemia is reached slowly, very high levels of potassium can be tolerated with no great problem. At the other end of the scale, once patients reach a potassium level of 2.5, they will feel very weak indeed.

60. A full-time, rather overweight gardener of 53 years asks his GP to check his blood pressure as he is sure it is raised. Asked why he thinks so, he says that every time he bends down to pull out a weed he goes red in the face and feels dizzy. His BP is 130/80. What is the most likely explanation for this phenomenon?

This is a frequent complaint and is almost universally perceived as a symptom of 'blood pressure'. It is very difficult to convince patients that a raised blood pressure is, almost always, asymptomatic. It is not unusual to see people present at a check-up feeling perfectly well with a BP of 240/130, and yet if patients come in with a headache and their BP is 140/95 they will quite likely say, 'That explains it then'. It is not always the easiest thing in the world to convince them that the stress that is causing their headache might have put up their blood pressure a little. How often does the GP hear, in a week, 'Could you check my blood pressure, Doctor. I've had a bit of a headache'? Similarly, patients nearly always construe the invariably innocent spontaneous conjunctival haemorrhage as caused by blood pressure and probably heralding an imminent stroke.

I'm not sure that anybody has thought up an explanation for the phenomenon in this question. If my best guess is correct then a raised blood pressure could not be further from the truth. Might I suggest that, as the gardener bends over, his generous abdomen is squeezing his thorax and, in effect, produces a Valsalva manoeuvre. This results in a drop in blood pressure (probably causing the dizziness on standing), followed by a rise in blood pressure. Also, during, and for a little while after the Valsalva, the pulse rate slows further, contributing to the dizziness. The face goes red simply because of blood rushing down under the effect of gravity when the man bends over.

1. **A man of 57 suffers from moderately severe hypertension which is well controlled by the medication he receives. His wife uses salt in cooking and he occasionally adds extra salt to the food he is eating. He does not like salt substitutes. Is his GP justified in pressing him to change his dietary habits?**

No. The problem with salt is, quite simply, that to make any difference to the blood pressure the food has to have so little salt in it that it is really abysmal and completely tasteless.

There is a group of stoical, if not masochistic, subjects who will pursue such a diet, and they will show that with no salt at all the systolic and diastolic pressures will drop by about 10%. But in people who reduce the amount of salt in their diet by what would seem a sensible amount – no added salt, etc. – there is no significant fall in blood pressure. If you do persuade such patients to take up a completely salt-free diet they tend to go around the bend, because it's awful! And remember, virtually every prepared food you buy has some salt content.

In any event it is more than likely that such a person, mentioned in the question, is on a diuretic anyway and is getting rid of his excess sodium in comfort. One of the arguments for putting people with high cholesterols on cholesterol-lowering drugs is that they can, at least, go through what might turn out to be a foreshortened life eating decent food.

Having said all the above, there is one situation in which I do press for salt restriction – in cases of Afro-Caribbeans with hypertension (see Question 96).

62. Under what circumstances is it thought that diuretics and beta-blockers might increase the risk from ischaemic heart disease? Is there much evidence to suggest that they can?

There is no doubt that there is a small risk with both thiazide diuretics and certain beta-blockers of increasing the cholesterol and the triglyceride and, most importantly, increasing the level of low-density lipoprotein. We have to take some notice of this, as a 1% drop in cholesterol equals a 2% drop in mortality rate for the patient.

The changes, however, can be very, very small and when the patients are happy on their medication it isn't something I would rush in and change. If, however, I had a patient who had a cholesterol of greater than 7.5, an LDL of 6 or more and an HDL/LDL ratio of less than 0.2, I would try and avoid such drugs that might adversely affect the lipids.

These considerations affect my prescribing for new patients to some degree. If I was giving a beta-blocker to a new patient I would tend to give one that was water-soluble, rather than lipid-soluble, as it would have less effect on the patient's lipids. Modern beta-blockers also seem to have less effect on the lipids. In many hypertensives, in whom I previously used beta-blockers, I would now use ACE inhibitors. ACE inhibitors either have no effect on a patient's lipid status or they tend to improve it. Certainly many patients will say that they feel better on ACE inhibitors than they do on beta-blockers.

Arrythmias

3. **The mother of a 9-year-old child comes to see you. The child has distressing attacks of tachycardia. A diagnosis of Wolff-Parkinson-White syndrome has been made. The mother is upset because the possibility of surgery has been raised. Is this a treatment that is often required before the situation in WPW can be controlled? Is surgical treatment usually successful?**

Wolff-Parkinson-White syndrome is a congenital condition caused by an abnormal myocardial conductive tissue link between atrium and ventricle. During normal rhythm there can be a sudden electrical activity across this connection, from which a tachycardia can result.

The majority of people with Wolff-Parkinson-White syndrome do not have tachycardia at all. Of the remainder, most will be easily controlled by tablets. You are only talking about a tiny minority where you have to do any more in the way of treatment.

The operations are surprisingly successful. You either ablate the bypass tract or the bundle of His at operation, by cutting the offending tissue with a knife or, using a catheter, fry, freeze or electrically shock it. The success rate for such treatments is high, although sometimes the procedure has to be repeated.

4. **A doctor sees a very healthy little boy at his 3½-year medical. He notices that there seems to be some kind of cardiac irregularity in the form of extra beats. He refers the toddler to the cardiologist who says that they are atrial ectopics and should present no problem. Can the mother be totally reassured? Are the ectopics likely to disappear and, if so, when? Should the child be treated any differently from any other child in circumstances such as having an anaesthetic, etc?**

The mother should be totally reassured. In this context atrial ectopics are always totally innocent. The only situation in which ectopics might presage trouble is in the post-MI case or in the elderly, where they can precede atrial fibrillation.

In the child they are always benign and are accounted for by high vagal

53

tone. The vagus inhibits the sino-atrial node and high vagal tone results in ectopics and junctional ectopics. They may appear at any time from the toddler to the late teens, but tend to disappear as the child gets older. Children with high vagal tone also tend to be 'fainters'. This might lead to the unfortunate picture of a child 'with something wrong with his heart who passes out', which sounds a lot less benign than it actually is.

Fit young people tend to have high vagal tone. This is why you will see so many faints in a blood transfusion session done at the army barracks. High vagal tone can be of advantage because of its tendency to produce a slow pulse, which allows for a high level of pulse reserve on exercise.

65. A woman of 56 has fairly frequent attacks of some kind of arrhythmia. She is fixed up with a 24-hour monitor by the hospital on three occasions but she does not have an attack during the period of monitoring. She knows by her symptoms when she is having an arrrhythmia. There is a waiting list for the equipment. Short of taking her into hospital and keeping her continually monitored until she has an attack, is there anything else that can be done?

The only effective way of getting a recording in this case is for the lady to make the recording herself. There are two devices available. One is applied directly to the chest and records for a minute. This recording can then be sent down the telephone line for the cardiologist to diagnose.

The other device used is a form of black box, a small simplified portable electrocardiograph. The patient puts an electrode from the machine around each wrist as soon as she feels an arrhythmia coming on and a 15-minute-long reading can be taken.

In the present changing circumstances of GP funding and finances it will soon be possible for such readings to be played into the GP's computer, by means of a relatively simple electronic device, giving him or her an immediate ECG of the patient's problem and possibly making a long, tedious and expensive hospital referral and investigation unnecessary.

6. A retired dentist of 83 who has atrial fibrillation, which is both idiopathic and untroublesome and has been present since he was 70, is visited at home. The man is seated and looks quite well. He is fibrillating with a pulse rate of 80/minute. He has no ankle oedema. When asked about his medication he walks a few yards in to the kitchen to find his pills (digoxin 125 microgrammes daily). When he returns he is breathless with a pulse rate of 150/min. Should the doctor take any action?

Yes. Many patients have a difficulty with atrial fibrillation in which the heart rate is controlled at rest but not with exercise. And, sometimes, the problem can arise with very little exercise indeed. The pulse rate might be quite normal but, within a minute or two of starting to walk, can shoot up to 200/min. This can produce marked breathlessness, irrespective of anything to do with the left ventricle or concurrent LVF.

In this kind of case another anti-arrhythmic has to be used but it isn't always a situation easy to control. Amiodarone is the best drug, in this context, by a mile. It does however have a number of side effects. The other drugs to consider are flecainide, verapamil or a beta-blocker, but these can only be used if there is no substantial left ventricular dysfunction, otherwise they might encourage the onset of failure.

When seeing a patient who is fibrillating, with a relatively normal rate, but who complains of breathlessness on effort, it might be worthwhile for the doctor to get the patient to walk a few paces and see if the pulse rate does go up dramatically.

Ideally, a patient presenting with the kind of problem described above should be referred to a cardiologist, because some kind of monitoring will almost certainly be required.

7. A GP is told that the old age pensioner he sent into hospital the previous night has been fixed up with a temporary pacemaker. How, and under what circumstances, are they fitted? How temporary are they and are they generally used in combination with anti-arrhythmic therapy?

A pacemaker will be put in for a persistent bradycardia of, say, anything less than 50. I'm speaking here of the generally unwell person rather than the super athlete! There are two reasons for this. Firstly, if the heart continues at that rate the patient will gradually go into failure, and secondly, the patient is at risk from having a Stokes-Adams attack which may result in death or significant cerebral damage.

In the elderly, 90% of such bradycardias are not due to severe coronary disease but are the consequence of some scarring in the Bundle of His. A 70-year-old man has an average life expectancy of 7 or 8 years. If you put a permanent pacemaker in such a patient, things work very well because the lithium cell lasts just about the same length of time. A convenient arrangement . . . though of course replacement is possible in the man whose shelf life is longer than his battery.

If a patient with severe bradycardia was picked up in outpatients or casualty you would put in a temporary pacemaker straight away before arranging a permanent pacemaker. The pacemaker lead is put in through the neck down into the tip of the right ventricle. The pacemaker box is worn externally.

As soon as that had been done you would ring up the regional unit to arrange transfer of the patient to be fitted up with a permanent pacemaker, The temporary pacemaker can be left in for up to ten days, but the longer it is left in the more likely complications, such as infection, are likely to arise. The sooner the permanent pacemaker is put in the better.

Some patients experience both slow and fast heart rates. At one end they need the pacemaker and at the other anti-arrhymics. The two treatments are completely compatible. As a general rule pacemakers are remarkably reliable.

68. A man of 50 gets recurrent attacks of tachycardia. He takes anti-arrhythmic drugs but these are not always successful . . . neither does he like taking such medication because of the side effects he encounters. He says that his brother in the USA has a similar problem but has been fitted with a device that slows down his heart. Is this possible?

I wouldn't like to have to pay his brother's medical bill. We are talking Megabucks. There are such devices fitted like permanent pacemakers which can sense tachycardias, and when alerted they send a minute shock back down the wire, into the ventricle, and revert the patient into sinus rhythm.

Even more exciting are those that can sense ventricular fibrillation and do the same thing. A very good idea. The only snag, of course, is the cost. Such pacemaker/intrinsic defibrillators cost in the region of £20,000. They are not needed often but they can be very useful if anti-arrhythmics are not working.

9. An apparently very fit man of 48 who has prolonged and frequent exercise is said, in a report from a works medical, to have a 'degree of heart block' on his ECG. Is it necessarily significant and, if so, why?

There are three degrees of heart block that can be shown on an ECG:

1) First-degree heart block which is, simply, represented by a long PR interval.

2) Second-degree heart block where there is either an increasingly long PR interval until the P wave drops a QRS complex (Wenckebach), or 2 to 1 block in which there are two P waves to every QRS.

3) Third-degree block, or complete heart block where there is no association at all between the QRS complexes and the P waves.

The athletic heart is associated with first degree block quite frequently, sometimes with Wenckebach block and, very occasionally, with 2 to 1 block, but never with complete heart block.

The athletic heart, as the man above may well have, can present great problems of diagnosis. There is less concern when the patient you are assessing is twenty-five years old, but at forty-plus you are never quite sure what you are dealing with.

In the athletic, supernormal, heart you may find left bundle branch block, right bundle branch block, left ventricular hypertrophy, right ventricular hypertrophy, slowing of the SA node with junctional rhythms occasionally occurring and, sometimes, such bradycardias that when the person is asleep and breathing deeply the heart may not beat for two or three seconds at a time. All this in people who are particularly fit.

It is extremely difficult looking at routine ECGs from such annual medicals as mentioned in the question, without the benefit of seeing the patient, to know whether you are dealing with an abnormal heart or a supernormal heart. First-degree heart block may well represent cardiac ill-health in an unfit, 48-year-old smoker with a raised cholesterol.

Sometimes, the only way to sort out these problems, after examining the patient and taking a careful history to exclude chest pain, is to carry out a formal exercise test under proper, supervised conditions and see how he or she performs.

The person with third-degree block needs a pacemaker (see Question 67).

70. **A man of 70 who is normally in very good health complains of a cough and feeling breathless. His wife has just had a chest infection. He appears to have caught the infection but is also found to be fibrillating at a rate of 120/min. Is the bronchitis a likely cause of the fibrillation? Is the fibrillation likely to go by itself when the chest infection settles? Should digitalis therapy be started straight away?**

The bronchitis is a very likely cause of the fibrillation. Fibrillation in a 70-year-old can be precipitated by a large number of things, a shaking-up of the body in some way. A chest infection in this context is very common.

When the chest infection has gone there is a very fair chance, better than 50%, that the rhythm will revert to normal. I would treat this man with digoxin simply because the pulse rate is rather fast and might cause him some cardiac embarrassment. Digoxin will slow down the rate; it would not necessarily cardiovert him, but that doesn't matter. You are just after a slower rate and the man would feel more comfortable.

I probably wouldn't treat with digoxin if his pulse rate was a hundred or below. I wouldn't digitalise him in the old sense of giving initial loading doses, I would just start him on a dose of digoxin 125 micrograms daily. After all, digoxin is not really an emergency drug for arrhythmia. In an emergency situation you would use amiodarone.

If the man stopped fibrillating as his chest infection got better, I would take him off the digoxin and with a bit of luck he wouldn't fibrillate again. If the man continued fibrillating, anticoagulants might be considered (see Question 19). Indeed, with this man, I might well consider starting him on daily aspirin even if he did stop fibrillating.

71. **A chartered accountant of 68 years complains that, on some days, he feels as though his heart is going to stop. On being questioned further it sounds as though he is having ventricular ectopics, and examination confirms this. Should either the doctor or the patient be alarmed and should either do anything about it? What if the man is found to have asymptomatic mitral regurgitation?**

Ventricular ectopics are astonishingly common. The incidence is roughly proportional to the age of the patient. Approximately 30% of 30-year-olds have ventricular ectopics as do 40% of 40-year-olds. They can be found, to a greater or lesser extent, on routine 24-hour monitoring. The incidence rises to 100% in 70-year-olds. The condition is almost invariably benign.

Very rarely do such ectopics represent any heart disease at all. Even if you get two ectopics together, which theoretically constitutes VT, it is nearly always benign.

The classic way to be absolutely sure of this is to get the patient to exercise. If the ectopics disappear then they are definitely benign. Even if they continue with exercise they are, quite often, also benign.

Patients with mitral incompetence, particularly if related to mitral leaflet syndrome, can have an enormous incidence of ectopics, sometimes said to be 100%. Clearly, in this situation, there are problems because the ectopics are frequent and perceived a great deal.

And there's the rub. The problem with ectopics, as with those that upset the chap above, is when they are perceived. In such cases they can make people frightened and destroy their quality of life, and should be treated. The best treatment is a beta-blocker. If patients are unable to take a beta-blocker because of asthma, the alternatives are verapamil or flecainide.

2. A rather anxious student of 19 suffers from attacks of palpitations. She is mildly asthmatic. The attacks usually last for half an hour or so. When she attends the hospital nothing abnormal is found, and on two occasions she is fitted up with a 24-hour monitor but no attack is recorded. How far would you be justified in investigating and treating a person with this background and history?

The second sentence of the question absolutely excludes the use of a beta-blocker, so we have to take it from there.

We are talking about a 19-year-old girl, so the chances that she has anything wrong with her heart outside of congenital disease are virtually nil. If she did have any congenital heart disease it would have shown up by now. Therefore, whatever palpitations she may have, there is no danger.

With an SVT, which this will almost certainly be, she could go on with a heart rate of 200 for a couple of weeks without any bother. So there is no worry about the heart itself. It is the palpitations that upset her. As the palpitations are supraventricular, anti-arrhythmics will not have that much effect.

Until a few years ago, before they had 'earned' their current opprobrium, benzodiazepines were considered by many doctors to be a most useful drug in this situation. With little in the way of side effects, they would calm down the patient and remove the stress that might well be causing the palpitations in the first place. Above all, having prescribed them successfully, in the short term one was able to say, 'This was only a mild tranquilliser. It made you better. It certainly wouldn't have done if you had any significant heart disease.' The patients, reassured, after a short course could be left with a few chlordiazepoxide, or whatever, so that if the event occurred again they would have an immediate effective treatment. I accept that they would be inappropriate in the long term.

Two drugs that you can use without fear of getting in the tabloids are verapamil and flecainide. Both have a negative inotropic effect, so that the heart beats less forcefully and the palpitations are less noticeable. Two to three months on these drugs, gradually tailing off, is generally all that is required. Teaching her about Valsalva and other similar manoeuvres may be helpful.

If the palpitations continue and the patient continues to be anxious, and understandably so, you have no option but to do more and more 24-hour tapes, or the patient can be given an event monitor (Question 33), or she could attend the surgery or casualty during an attack to get an ECG there and then.

Exercise

3. It is well documented that such exercise as jogging can provoke a sudden cardiac death. How common is sudden cardiac death during or following isometric exercises – press-ups, pull-ups, etc. – in the person's own bedroom? Are these exercises, in fact, more dangerous?

Many people who decide to take some form of exercise have substantial ischaemic heart disease without being aware of it. This must include 50% of all males over the age of 50 years. They buy a tracksuit and a pair of trainers and feel invincible. In this context isometric exercises are as dangerous as jogging . . . in theory. In both activities there is a sudden raise in afterload with a consequent rapid increase of back pressure on to the ventricle.

It is a dicey situation. If there is some ischaemia, sudden strain could result in pain, which at least gives a warning, or in ventricular fibrillation which, unfortunately, does not.

Having said that, I feel that isometric exercises, though in my mind not a particularly good idea for the unfit, are probably safer for two reasons. Firstly, they are usually done in the warm environment of the bedroom, rather than jogging, which in inclement weather can involve the mischief-making combination of exercise and cold. Secondly, isometrics in the bedroom tends to be an individual exercise in which people can pace themselves and ease up if they feel a bit tired, as opposed to jogging where, if running with others, they might feel obliged to keep up even if they are getting distressed.

I think folk probably exercise much less hard at home than they do when jogging . . . there are a substantial number of jogging deaths but I have not come across one of a person dying whilst exercising at home.

However . . . exercise, generally, is very good for you. It appears to be cardioprotective (it improves the lipid profile) and even in those who have established IHD it can improve mobility, distance walked before angina, etc. In moderation, it seems beneficial to all systems of the body. What is inappropriate is sudden, severe exercise in the very unfit.

In my view the best exercise of all is fast walking i.e. 2 miles in less than 30 minutes two or three times a week. There is a huge difference between walking on the flat and walking up hill. For those who are fit and want to get fitter, I would recommend them to walk up a slope at their own pace, or go up and down the stairs a few dozen times each day.

74. A fit young man applies to join the army. He does judo twice a week and jogs five miles three times a week and also does weight training. He is a little over his 'ideal' weight for height and smokes ten cigarettes a day. On examination the army doctor says that his pulse recovery from exercise is slow. He does an ECG, which shows left ventricular hypertrophy. The man is rejected – and dejected. His GP refers him to the local cardiologist who investigates him further and says that there is nothing wrong with him. How can he tell?

Unfortunately, it is not uncommon for people to be labelled in this way. It often results from an ECG report being made with no reference to the particular circumstances of the patient. Let us look at this case in its various aspects.

To get it out of the way immediately, smoking ten cigarettes a day is not good for anybody but is unlikely, as yet, to have affected this man's heart. This is a young man who does a lot of exercise and he almost certainly has exercise-induced ventricular hypertrophy – the athletic heart. He has built up his cardiac biceps, as it were. He is said to be slightly overweight. He would have to be at least 30% overweight for it to have any particular bad effect on his heart. Nevertheless, you only have to look at diminutive Welsh fly-halves weighing 13½-stone to realise that the very fit, in whom muscle has replaced fat, can be heavy for their size. Muscle, volume for volume, is heavier than fat.

I suspect this man's pulse rate is generally slow. I might be concerned if the pulse rate did not fall below 100 within 5–6 minutes of exercise, but in the context of the medical he is probably very 'fired-up' anyway, and his pulse might take until he has got out of the building before it starts to come down.

The cardiologist can confirm that this man is just very fit by doing a treadmill exercise test, which will show up most things, and an echo which will show up the rest . . . particularly a HOCM.

75. A keen squash player of 38 is found to have a fairly classic pericarditis. It is presumed to be viral. As one of the commonest causes of pericarditis is myocardial infarction, how far should one go to exclude this?

You have to take these guys pretty seriously. Even if the pericarditis is viral he could still drop down dead by running around like an idiot ... a situation not entirely unknown amongst squash players. It must be remembered that a lot of people with a viral pericarditis have an underlying myocarditis as well. For this reason, and for the other possibility of infarction, I think all cases of pericarditis should be admitted to hospital to be sorted out.

In my humble opinion, squash is the daftest of games. When you have four grey walls around you you tend to go bananas. Aggression builds up and people will not stop trying to beat their opponent, however awful they may feel. There is this idea that you can 'sweat a virus out'. Some people do run around with myocarditis and, on occasion, drop down dead. The same phenomenon is found amongst the zealots of the jogging fraternity.

Sport is grand, the spice of life, enormously enjoyable, good for you. But do not run or play vigorous games when you are not well. It is silly, and dangerous.

76. A man of 47 suffers a myocardial infarction. He appears not to take the attack very seriously and is in a hurry to 'get back to normal as soon as possible and forget all about it'. He is offered help by the rehabilitation department of the local cardiology unit but turns it down. Is this a wise decision?

The purpose of a cardiac rehabilitation unit is, by physical, psychological and educational methods, to get the patient back to normal – and back to regarding himself as normal – thereby restoring his confidence as soon as possible. This man appears to be achieving this end on his own and shouldn't be made to feel too guilty about turning down the formalised unit. Over three years those patients who have attended a coronary rehabilitation unit demonstrate a 20% reduction in mortality, compared to those who haven't. In a case like this, in which the man very much wants to get on with his life, I would let him do just that.

77. **Christmas Day. The fifty-year-old husband and wife look out of the window and see a very festive sight. Which of them should shovel the snow off the drive?**

There is an increased death rate in shovelling snow in cold weather, and at this age the husband is much more at risk than the wife. At the age of 50 a woman is still, most likely, protected by her hormones, and probably no more than 5% of women of this age will have significant atheroma. I suspect that at least 50% percent of men of this age have significant coronary artery narrowing.

The answer is, therefore, that the husband should sit down, have a Scotch, send his wife out (well wrapped up of course) and not worry.

Once the woman is past the menopause, however, the roles become reversed. Unless she is on HRT her cardiovascular risk will approximate to that of her husband. She could well, in addition, have some osteoporosis, making it more likely that she will fracture an arm or leg if she slips over.

A survey of snow-shovelling deaths (I believe it was carried out in Canada) showed that there is an increased sudden cardiac death rate during snow falls that require the shovelling treatment. However, taken over a period of two or three months the death rate is not above the average for less snowy years, rather suggesting that the people who dropped down, shovel in hand, were due to drop down anyway and this extra effort was just the precipitating factor in an inevitable and imminent process.

Cold and exercise are bad companions for ischaemic heart disease. Do not join a Christmas Day swim club if you have angina.

78. **A woman of 35, determined to lose weight, goes on a strict diet and takes a lot of vigorous exercise. She comes to the doctor because she has felt unwell, has had attacks of palpitations and, to cap it all, a 'friend' has told her that a female pop star died under similar circumstances. Is there an intrinsic danger in dieting and exercising at the same time, i.e. can hypoglycaemia contribute to acute cardiological situations such as arrhythmias?**

I do not know whether or not there is an official association between hypoglycaemia and sudden cardiac death, but I don't see why there should not be for a number of reasons.

There is an association between hypoglycaemia and sudden death in infants. It is one of the many factors involved in this complex and tragic situation that is not yet, in any way, fully understood. Neither are all the sudden cardiac deaths that occur during exercise easily explained. The vast majority must have an arrhythmic basic – certainly at the end!

A potent cause of arrhythmia is catecholamine release. Hypoglycaemia is associated with increased adrenaline production as the body attempts to mobilise more glucose. This extra adrenaline gives rise to the typical hypoglycaemic symptoms of dry mouth, sweating, tremor ... and palpitations.

It would be fair to say that extreme dieting and exercise could be a pretty dangerous mixture, particularly for a person who might already have some cardiac irritability resulting from atheroma, smoking, oral contraceptives, etc.

Unfortunately, most members of the general public consider exercise as effective a way of losing weight as dieting. It is not. It takes 20 miles of walking to work off a slice or two of bread. It is much easier to eat less bread. That is not to say that regular, moderate exercise, such as fast walking, is not an excellent accompaniment to a reasonable diet. The two are complimentary. But a 50-year-old man, 15 stones in weight, 5ft. 5in. tall, jogging until the sweat pours, or trying to keep up with the 20-year-olds at an aerobics class, does not bear thinking about.

Diet reasonably. Exercise reasonably.

One last thought. I have been thinking here about people who are overweight. Even more at risk are those fairly anorexic people who wish to become even more skeletal and use appetite suppressants, and even thyroxine, totally contraindicated in the euthyroid, to shed those last few grams of fat. The cardiac irritability in such people must be pretty intense, and violent exercise for them could certainly be lethal.

9. A mother consults you about her 6ft. 6in. basket-ball playing son. He has very tall parents and is nearly 16 years old. She has read about a famous player dropping down dead and asks you about Marfan's syndrome. What action can you take and how easy is the diagnosis to establish in marginal cases?

Marfan's cases drop dead for two reasons. Either they rupture a valve – aortic, or mitral – or they dissect the aorta, sometimes rupturing into the pericardium. In suspected Marfan's you must do an echocardiogram, particularly with reference to the aortic root size. If it is enlarging on serial echoes, on an annual basis, then it is likely to be Marfan's.

If the person has a true Marfan's syndrome you will, of course, get other signs such as hypermobility of joints, dislocation of lens, etc. Problems arise with a *forme fruste* Marfan's, which is a kind of half and half situation. The skeletal and other abnormalities are absent but the cardiac ones, and their associated risk, are not. In a case like this, therefore, of a very tall boy with no other stigmata of Marfan's I would think it worth doing an echocardiogram ... and similarly with any other abnormally tall young people.

Age, Risk and Prognosis

80. How do you regard moderate obesity, e.g. the 5ft. 9in., 14-stone man in the assessment of cardiac risk? Do you differentiate the risk differently between men and women?

The answer is that mild obesity, even moderate obesity, represents only a very small cardiac risk on its own. You have to be about 30% above your 'ideal weight' before the cardiac risk is measurably increased, which makes something of a nonsense of these 'weigh 'em, measure 'em' schemes much beloved by the present Department of Health. You have to be visibly fat to be at risk.

Obesity is more significant in men as a risk factor, because women are protected by their hormones. Women, indeed, unless grossly overweight, do not seem to be at much risk at all from obesity.

Being fat, from a lot of other points of view, is not a very good idea. You are slower and there is more wear and tear on the joints and muscles. If ischaemic heart disease is already established and you are obese, it can be very beneficial to lose some weight because you will be able to exercise longer before you get angina, and you will feel generally much better.

81. A man of 56 returns from the hospital outpatients. The senior house officer has told him that he has 'a cardiomyopathy' but has not told him what it is in terms that the poor man can understand. How would you explain the condition to him in such a way that he would not immediately go out and throw himself off a bridge?

The most important thing in a case like this, as it is in so much prognostic medicine, is the choice of phraseology. It is the old story of the bottle being half full rather than half empty. If you say that the pumping muscle of his heart is weakened and not pumping properly then you will worry him. What I would say to the man is that the muscle is not being as vigorous as it should be and that it needs to be helped. I would say that we could help the situation with medication and that is what we are going to do.

Cardiomyopathy is certainly not all doom and gloom. It depends upon the circumstances. It is true that some cardiomyopathic hearts can return to being reasonably normal, particularly those with cardiomyopathy following a virus infection. The same is true of alcoholic cardiomyopathy if the person stops drinking. It is not a death sentence, by a long way. Even if they don't improve, some cardiomyopathies stay at a very stable level for a number of years.

The severity of a cardiomyopathy can be determined on echocardiograph by measuring the ventricular diameter in systole and diastole. The normal diastolic diameter is 5 cm, going down to 3 cm in systole. Once you get a situation of the diameter going down from 7 cm to 6 cm – enlarged and hardly moving – the patient should be dissuaded from joining the Christmas Club. Locally, in our simple way, we call this 7 and 6 measurement a 'dog licence' (7/6d in old money). Beyond a dog licence – 8 to 7, or 9 to 8 – is definitely bad news. 7 to 5, or 7 to 4 as you might get in hypertensive enlargement of the left ventricle, is nothing to be pleased about (see Question 37) but it does represent a much better prognostic group.

It is the patients who have a large, very poorly contracting ventricle who make the bulk of those who receive heart transplants.

For patients with cardiomyopathy, however, the great advance medically has been the appearance of the ACE inhibitors. Both the life expectancy and the quality of life have been improved by these drugs.

So the story is not all bad. There is a lot that can be done. Some cardomyopathies improve by themselves, moderately severe cases can be dramatically helped with diuretics, digoxin and ACE inhibitors, and the most serious may be amenable to transplant, an effective and increasingly common operation.

82. A man of 54 has an MI. He recovers well and is discharged from hospital after a few days. He comes to his GP's surgery and says that he is surprised that he has been given no other medication than 150 mgm aspirin a day. What drugs might he have been given that could improve his prognosis?

In some units no other drugs would be given routinely. It depends upon the preferences of the consultant concerned. In our hospital, if there is no contra-indication, we start a beta-blocker, such as atenolol 50 mgm daily, on Day One and continue for one year. The contraindications to this treatment include the usual ones to beta-blockers, such as bronchospasm. In the context of post-MI, however, heart failure is the main reason for withholding this group of drugs.

If given, the beta-blockers confer a 25% improvement in survival for the first year, so they are well worth the effort. Unfortunately, many of the patients don't tolerate them for a variety of reasons ranging from impotence to 'beta-blocker blues'.

The ACE inhibitors have less side effects than beta-blockers and are known to improve prognosis in the post-MI patient with failure. There is not, however, for the ACE inhibitors, the same weight of evidence that supports the beta-blockers in the context of the asymptomatic patient. Nevertheless they are very good drugs in heart failure and appear to extend life expectancy. If the post-MI patient, therefore, has a sniff of failure about him it is worth giving an ACE. In overt failure, an ACE inhibitor would be an absolute drug of choice.

Although many post-MI patients do have arrhythmias, such as ventricular ectopics, there is no point in giving anti-arrhythmics routinely after an infarct as they really give no improvement in prognosis. In the asymptomatic post-MI patient, calcium antagonists are not beneficial; indeed, the contrary may be true.

The recent ISIS 4 study showed that there was no evidence to support the use of magnesium or nitrates (other than those required to treat symptoms) following a heart attack. I would not use lipid-reducing drugs, in this context, if the cholesterol was below 6.5. I would think hard between 6.5 and 7.8, but would use them if the cholesterol was 8 or over.

33. A fit, active accountant of 72, still working full-time, has an MI on the golf course. His doctor phones up the local hospital and is told that as the man is over 70 he will be admitted under the geriatricians. His GP tries to insist that he be admitted under the cardiologist but is told, by an administrator, that it is hospital policy to admit all medical patients over the age of 70 under the geriatricians. Is this as clinically inappropriate as it is ludicrous?

It is ludicrous but, with reasonable co-operation, should not be clinically inappropriate.

Look at pictures of your grandfathers and grandmothers, or their parents, fifty and more years ago. Most people of 55 years were quite old then, and many of 70 years were very old. The world changes, not least in the expectation that people have to remain healthier for longer. And quite rightly so from a cardiological point of view.

I would happily recommend biologically healthy octogenarians for aortic valve replacement or CABG – or both if it came to that. In the USA, many people over the age of ninety have had these operations. I certainly think there should be virtually no age limit for angioplasty in the appropriate, symptomatic patient.

In this particular case the man should be treated the same, whoever admits him, and unless there is a contraindication he should be given some form of clot-busting therapy. In the early days of streptokinase and the like there was an initial reluctance to use such therapy in older patients, but all the evidence now suggests that it is the older patients who benefit most of all.

Though there should be no difference in management of the acute attack, there might be some difference in attitude at follow-up. If the patient recovers well I suspect that the attitude of the geriatrician would be to let sleeping dogs lie, whereas I feel that the cardiologist might be a lot more aggressive in his attempts to try and prevent further trouble. The GP, if he wishes and feels it would be appropriate, can always transfer the patient, following discharge from hospital, from geriatrician to cardiologist in the outpatient setting where there is no division by age. Happily, some geriatricians will do this themselves if they feel that a particular patient requires more cardiological assessment.

84. An elderly lady has severe, chronic congestive cardiac failure. She has been somewhat breathless at rest for a long time and takes a full spectrum of medication, including diuretics and ACE inhibitors. Her son wants to go for a much needed holiday. He asks his GP whether his mother is likely to get worse, or even die, in the next two weeks. Are there any features of CCF which might suggest an imminent demise?

The prognosis of an elderly patient in heart failure poses a very difficult question that is impossible to answer although, for one reason or another, it is often asked.

People who die of heart failure usually die in one of two ways. They either have a sudden arrhythmia, without any warning, or a gradual demise of death by drowning from pulmonary oedema, as predictable as the former is unpredictable.

If the old lady was gasping for breath at rest and waking several times in the night with paroxysmal, nocturnal dyspnoea, you would be justified in telling the son to think about delaying his holiday. If, on the other hand, she was breathless on minor effort and just able to get around, and had been the same for weeks or months, the son could be reassured that she might well go on for weeks, or months . . . or years. He should take his well-earned rest.

As I intimated, some of these old people with severe heart failure can go on for years. The prognostic aspect not only involves their children's holidays but, more commonly, decisions that regard the management of other illnesses they might have. Their possible long-term survival may have a bearing on whether they have other treatments such as cataract operations, joint replacements or even major cancer surgery, and it is in these circumstances that the cardiologist's opinion is most often sought . . . an opinion that might be no less chancey or scientifically-based than the tipster's 3.30 at Newmarket.

85. A man of 47 has a myocardial infarction. The GP sends for an ambulance. The wife asks, 'He will be all right, won't he Doctor?' The man has little more than an ache in the chest but is sweating profusely and has a low blood pressure. Is this a worse prognostic picture than if the man had a much more severe pain without sweating or hypotension?

In the case described above there are two possible diagnoses. In the first the man is scared stiff by his heart attack, and consequently is in a state of great vagal stimulation leading to faintness, sweating and pallor. The other possibility is that he is in cardiogenic shock, where his grossly damaged heart is failing rapidly.

I think that in this case, in the early stage of an infarct, the former is more likely. As long as the man did not have a tachycardia, a shot of atropine given in this situation could make him feel much better. Myocardial infarction is a dynamic process and it is not usually until quite late in the day, some hours after the initial attack, that the myocardium is sufficiently damaged for the patient to go into cardiogenic shock. It is theoretically possible to infarct so severely that cardiogenic shock can appear very early, but it is the exception rather than the rule.

The absence of sweating does not mean that the person is not having a myocardial infarct. There is no relationship between pain and prognosis in myocardial infarction. Possibly as many as 20% of infarctions are painless . . . particularly in diabetics.

86. In your opinion, which age of man most determines his outlook from the point of view of heart disease – (a) conception, (b) 0–20 years, (c) 20–40 years, or (d) 50 years?

The conception part is, of course, most important. You have to choose your parents most carefully, both from the point of view of developing heart disease and of being more than averagely prone to diabetes. These are very strong genetic factors.

The 0 to 20 year period I feel is most important in the development of habits, good or bad. Are you going to smoke, eat fish and chips seven times a week, drink large amounts of alcohol, be a couch potato? You probably decide on your mode of living before your twentieth birthday. The same may be said about salt consumption, although as I have remarked in Question 61, I think this is a minimal problem. The most important of these factors is smoking. If you don't smoke in your first twenty years then you probably never will.

The period 20 to 40 years decides on how much stress you are going to live under. The habits developed before 20 can – and, under stress – will worsen. Such a man under stress can, typically, smoke forty cigarettes a day, eat massively when he gets home, have a lot to drink in an effort to relax, and take no exercise.

At 50 years you will have most of the atheroma you are going to get and by this time it is too late to alter things very dramatically. A change in life style will help somewhat, but not nearly as much as action taken a long time before. Stopping smoking at this age will reduce risk, but never back to the non-smoker's level. It is unlikely that dietary change alone will reduce any established atheroma, although modern lipid-lowering drugs might have some effect. Exercise can improve the lipid profile, particularly by increasing the HDL. I discuss the question of cholesterol lowering with regard to primary and secondary prevention of ischaemic heart disease in Question 93.

Major Procedures

87. For what kind of patient, with what kind of illness, is heart transplant now considered the treatment of choice? Is it sufficiently available that a GP should have it at the back of his mind when discussing a patient's treatment?

Heart transplant is a very good operation. In our district (East Berkshire, approximate population 350,000) in the past twelve years there have been ten heart transplants carried out on our patients, *all* of whom, at the time of writing, are still alive. Three-year survival has been given at 80%, and I suspect much the same survival rate applies at 4 and 5 years.

It is a treatment that GPs should consider. For example, if a person under the age of 55, in spite of medication, is more or less breathless at rest from heart failure due to a poorly functioning myocardium, heart transplant is probably the treatment of choice . . . indeed probably the only treatment.

There are almost certainly enough hearts to go around. About 400 transplants are done a year in the UK and there are now more than 1000 recipients alive.

88. A psychiatrist friend tells you that he has been offered the choice of an angioplasty or a bypass for his coronary artery blockage. The surgeon has made this concession because of your friend's professional status. In the present state of the art which would you advise, and why?

It is possible that your psychiatrist friend has got hold of the wrong end of the stick. There is usually no question of choice. If the coronary artery lesion was amenable to angioplasty this is what, in the first event, he would most likely be offered. It is not an operation. It is particularly suitable for a lesion near the origin of an artery. You can't do an angioplasty where there are multiple lesions a long way down the artery. In these circumstances only a coronary artery bypass would be suitable.

Two-thirds of patients who have an angioplasty only need to have it done once to achieve a successful result, that is, a 90% chance of freedom from angina at six months. The rest need it repeated, usually within the first three months. Two years after angioplasty, however, angina will have recurred, though perhaps not as severely as before, in 50% of patients. Recurrence of angina is much less common and longer delayed in those who have had a CABG.

If there was an equivocal situation, in which either procedure could be used, it would be a toss-up between the considerably less trauma of the angioplasty compared to the better result given by the CABG.

In the right circumstances – left main stem disease or triple artery disease – CABG confers a percentage improvement in life expectancy. Angioplasty, not suitable for, nor indicated for ischaemic heart disease of this severity, is used to treat symptoms. It does not improve life expectancy.

89. **A patient tells you that his cousin suffered a heart attack, was rushed into a cardiothoracic surgical unit and had an operation that 'saved his life'. What is the likely explanation for this story? Are there any circumstances in which the GP should be phoning up the heart surgeon and not the cardiologist?**

There are a number of possibilities here. He could have ruptured something, either the cusp of a mitral valve or the intraventricular septum. Either way he would have gone rapidly into heart failure and would have needed urgent surgical intervention. Ideally surgery would have been delayed for six weeks after the attack, but if he was going rapidly into severe failure it would have been required straight away.

Another reason for operating straight away could have been to unblock a coronary artery where the patient's blood pressure was extremely low and he was in cardiogenic shock. Occasionally you can open up patients like this, unblock the artery and restore function. This situation is called a 'stunned myocardium', where the myocardium is very ischaemic and not working but comes back to life again when the blood flow is restored.

The most likely explanation for the story above is that the patient did not actually have a heart attack, i.e. a myocardial infarction, but an attack of crescendo angina. Patients often call all kinds of things 'heart attacks' when they are not strictly so. It may well be – particularly if the patient had already been investigated by angiogram and was on the waiting list for surgery – that the surgeon decided, in view of the crescendo angina, that it was a good idea to perform a CABG as a matter of urgency in the hope of preventing an infarction.

In an ideal world all patients with crescendo angina should be investigated as soon as possible, and if angiography demonstrates a significant lesion they should have an angioplasty or CABG without delay. As it is, financial constraints mean that the patient goes on a long waiting list for investigation and, after that has been done, goes on another long waiting list for surgery. No amount of money spent on administration will overcome that.

0. You are present at a party when a man of 53 drops to the floor with a cardiac arrest. You give resuscitation but do not appear to be making any headway. You think about giving the man intracardiac adrenaline on the assumption that there is nothing to lose. Might this assumption be incorrect? Might it increase the chances of the patient surviving to 'enjoy' severe brain damage?

Resuscitation in these circumstances, properly administered, can keep a patient in reasonable shape for up to an hour, that is to say, recoverable. You will need someone to help you as it is impossible to keep up single-handed resuscitation for much more than twenty minutes.

Immediately you are called to the man you should ask someone to call an ambulance on 999. In all likelihood a properly equipped ambulance will be on the scene within minutes and, in most parts of the country, the patient will be in hospital not many minutes later, well before the hour is up.

To attempt intracardiac adrenaline at home may very well result in cardiac tamponade, killing what might have been a retrievable patient . . . and many people are resuscitated in what might seem like hopeless circumstances. If the patient does die of the tamponade, legal action may be taken against you.

Miscellaneous

91. **A man of 55 is having a work-out at a health club. Suddenly he gets a pain in his chest and also a pain in the left shoulder and arm, running down into his hand. He is taken to hospital where an MI is confirmed. He recovers very well and some weeks later an exercise test is reported on as being normal. Many months later he consults his GP because he still has the pain in his left arm and hand that he had at the time of the infarct. It is not made worse by effort. If anything, it seems worse at rest. How is this pain to be dealt with?**

Many years ago this was a commonly encountered phenomenon and was called the 'shoulder/hand syndrome'. The pain was often very severe and was thought to be due to the long periods of immobility, often six weeks or more of bed-rest, that was prescribed when a person had a coronary.

It is, in fact, most likely akin to Dressler's syndrome, an auto-immune antibody reaction. The treatment is entirely separate from the coronary and it should be treated, and regarded, as a musculo-skeletal problem. Physiotherapy, NSAIDs, manipulation and acupuncture can all be used, but sometimes the pain is most difficult to eradicate. It is very important to reassure the patient that it is *not* symptomatic of ongoing heart disease.

92. **A man with chronic heart failure who suffers from dyspnoea reminds you that his next-door neighbour, who has chronic obstructive airways disease, receives considerable benefit from continuous oxygen as supplied by a domestic oxygen exchange machine. He asks whether he, too, would benefit from such a device. Would he?**

Some patients with COAD benefit greatly from these machines. Oxygen is, after all, a bronchodilator and the oxygen in these circumstances serves to relieve some of the distress. Within reason, the more you have, the better you are and the longer you live ... and some of these breathless patients can go on for years and years.

There is no evidence, however, that oxygen prolongs life in chronic heart failure. Oxygen in heart failure is best used as an adjunct for someone who gets more breathless on occasion. There is no particular place for continuous oxygen, because most patients with chronic heart failure are not gasping at rest all the time like people with COAD. If they are breathless all the time, they are either not on sufficient medication or have such severe failure that their prognosis is extremely limited.

Nevertheless, I think that oxygen at home should be prescribed more often than it is for patients in failure. It is very comforting, both physically and psychologically, to have an oxygen cylinder by the bed if you suddenly become breathless.

93. Is there any evidence that making a radical change in an unhealthy life style might bring about a reversal in the process of arteriosclerosis? How strong is the evidence that fish oils have anything to offer in this direction?

For the first part of the question the answer is, officially, 'No'. But that can't stop conjecture. There is indeed no evidence, in the primary situation of a person having no proven heart disease, that the atheromatous process would be reversed by diet, cholesterol-lowering drugs, exercise, etc. Just imagine how difficult that would be to prove in the 'well' population.

However, there is evidence to suggest that dropping the cholesterol sufficiently, in people in a secondary situation – i.e. those who have had an infarct or are suffering from angina, intermittent claudication etc. – can reduce their atheroma by several per cent per annum. Now this is easy enough to show, because these people will be happy enough to have the investigations done which will demonstrate this to be the case. You can't, on the other hand, go up to a man in the street, with apparently nothing wrong with him, and ask if you can do one coronary angiogram on him now and another one in a year's time, following a twelve-months abstinence from fish and chips and eggs and bacon.

In secondary prevention it is very worthwhile using every device available to halt, or bring about regression in, the atheromatous process with such things as reasonable diet, reasonable exercise and cholesterol-lowering substances. Common sense, however, gives us every reason to suppose that if cholesterol lowering is beneficial in the people who are already ill, it must have some effect on the people who are heading that way.

Stopping smoking does have a beneficial effect on IHD prognosis but it takes some years to reach a substantial level. The effect of treating hypertension does not have a spectacular effect on reducing IHD, although it does of course reduce the amount of strokes. There is no great evidence that eating like an eskimo and filling up with fish oils has much effect on IHD or the lipids except by dropping the triglyceride a little. They may have some effect on clotting, but aspirin is by far the more effective drug in this context.

If I was eating a reasonable diet that was balanced and not excessive in its fat content, and I was having a reasonable amount of exercise, and was to find that I had a cholesterol of greater than 7.5 or an LDL above 6, I would seriously think about taking a statin or similar, because such drugs seem pretty safe, and lowering cholesterol from that level must be beneficial. I would still, however, insist on having butter with my new potatoes.

94. In what ways might AIDS present as a cardiological condition?

AIDS does not present as a cardiological condition. Cardiological problems in the disease, however, are not uncommon. There is a cardiological clinical component in about 10% of AIDS patients. At post-mortem about 50% of AIDS sufferers are found to have histological changes in the heart, most commonly myocarditis. The commonest clinical cardiological problem found in AIDS patients is a cardiomyopathy. You can also get myocarditis, pericarditis, endocarditis, arrhythmias, heart block . . . almost anything in the book. But not as a presenting feature. In this district I am asked to see about one AIDS case a month.

95. A young mother is very distressed to be told that her healthy young son of 1 year has a small VSD. What are the chances that it will close itself? Will the child need prophylactic antibiotics if dental or surgical treatments are considered . . . and until when?

If a child has a small VSD at 1 year the chance that it will have closed by the age of 5 is between 30% and 50%. Remember that the smaller the VSD, the louder the murmur and the more powerful the jet that will come through the defect from left to right. This jet can damage the right ventricular wall and it is in this area of damage that SBE can set up.

The child would certainly have to have prophylactic antibiotics, prior to surgical or dental procedures, until it was shown that the VSD had closed . . . or for the rest of his life. Closure is indicated by complete disappearance of the murmur and a normal Doppler echocardiogram.

96. A doctor, who has worked for many years in rural Somerset, comes to do a locum in West London. He finds the practice he is covering is comprised almost entirely of Asian and Afro-Caribbean patients. From a cardiovascular point of view, will he encounter unfamiliar disease patterns and will the treatments required differ from those in his usual practice?

There is no doubt that members of the Asian community present with coronary artery disease at a younger age, have larger infarcts, have more diabetes and have more complications of ischaemic heart disease than the Caucasian population. People with suspicious histories have to be taken very seriously, even at quite young ages, as ischaemic heart disease appears to occur, on average, ten years earlier than in the Caucasian population. Always be on the look-out for diabetes in Asian patients and test their urine frequently.

Afro-Caribbean patients very commonly develop hypertension, and that hypertension is very often serious and most difficult to treat. The hypertension very often responds much better to diuretics and calcium antagonists than it does to beta-blockers and ACE inhibitors – C and D rather than A and B. That having been said, the hypertension is often very difficult to treat and frequently requires four different hypotensive agents at a time.

This is the one group of patients to whom I do make a song and dance about the dietary sodium. Afro-Caribbeans tend to have a very high salt intake and this must be modified. Afro-Caribbeans have a lower incidence of myocardial infarction and a higher incidence of stroke than the general population.

97. A 76-year-old lady, recently widowed, lives in a country cottage one and a half miles from the nearest village. Because she had suffered from angina for the last five years her husband, prior to his death, had done all the driving. She now wishes to drive again and has been asked, by an insurance company, to attend her GP for a medical which will decide whether or not she is fit to drive. She tells her GP that she only needs the car to get to the local shop and her angina prevents her walking that far. She says that if she drives on main roads her angina is bad and if she drives on motorways she feels very ill indeed. Nevertheless there is a quiet country lane between her and the village and she promises to drive only on that route. The car is her lifeline. Is her GP justified in cutting it?

Unlike many neurological complaints, in the context of the DVLA, most cardiological contraindications to driving are relative. One question has to be asked. Is the condition bad enough to make driving hazardous to the driver and the public at large.

The GP cannot pass this lady as fit to drive. Angina in itself is not a contraindication to driving, as long as it is not provoked by driving. A person is either fit to drive or not fit to drive. It is a painful duty for the GP but it has to be faced. The same argument applies to all people with a relative disability, whether it be cardiological, neurological or whatever. That is – all roads or none at all. To be told that you cannot drive any more is very upsetting indeed. For this elderly lady it is a great blow against her personal freedom and a reminder of increasing dependency to come.

There is, however, a positive side to this situation and, once the nettle has been grasped, can give great relief. From an economic point of view she has a capital asset – the car – which she can sell, and she will no longer pay car tax, insurance, maintenance charges or have to buy petrol. All this releases a fair amount of money.

Many local taxi firms are often quite happy to make a regular arrangement with an elderly person to take them to their local shops, and the accumulated cost in a year may be less than what the car was costing. Also, in the country, there are often voluntary schemes to which, if she wished, she could make a contribution. It is worth saying to the lady that if she were taken ill at the wheel it might not just be herself who would be endangered. Ask her to imagine how she would feel if she ran into a young mother and her children.

One other alternative, perhaps ideal in this case, would be for her to have one of the little electric buggies, especially designed for the immobile elderly, that will take her down to the village. It should not upset her and even if she did become ill and lose control, would cause no great mayhem. She does not have to be passed fit to drive one of those.

8. **A man of 47 in generally good health wakes up in the night on two or three occasions with an aching pain in his lower central chest. He gets up, takes some of his wife's alginate and a couple of paracetamol and the pain soon goes. He mentions it to his doctor during a routine medical. His GP says that it is most likely oesophageal reflux with associated spasm and, unless it is more than occasional, of no concern. Is his GP correct in his reassurance.?**

I think he is. This is a common symptom although most reflux symptoms tend to occur just before you go to sleep. If this pain happens only once or twice I would reassure. However, on occasion, it represents coronary artery spasm which can give this kind of night pain.

It is worth trying GTN. It will of course relieve both oesophageal spasm and coronary artery spasm. Coronary artery spasm, however, tends to be relieved in seconds whereas oesophageal spasm may take up to ten minutes to respond.

Oesophageal spasm can also be relieved by drinking a very cold drink, or sucking an ice cube, or, some say, having a tot of neat whisky!

9. **Worried, by press reports of such tragedies, that his apparently very fit, sport-talented son of 14 years 'might drop down dead', a PE master persuades a doctor to arrange an echocardiogram for the boy. The echo shows hypertrophic obstructive cardiomyopathy. Would it have been best for all concerned not to have known?**

The answer is definitely 'No'. The boy and his family must know what is going on. Hypertrophic cardiomyopathy at this age can be very severe and can result very easily in the sudden death this man fears, particularly with exercise. There have been many reports of this kind of tragedy.

Very careful management is required if someone is found to have a HOCM. The severity of the condition needs to be assessed very accurately, not only with echocardiography but also with exercise test, 24-hour tape and even with coronary angiogram and biopsy of the left ventricular muscle. The patient has to be very, very carefully handled, ideally by a person who specialises in cardiomyopathy.

Great care has to be taken as the athletic heart, which might very well be found in the kind of person described above, can mimic hypertrophic cardiomyopathy, particularly on ECG. A young, asymptomatic, very active person whose ECG gives the appearance of 'the athletic heart' – large, left ventricular forces – should also have an echocardiogram to exclude hypertrophic myopathy. If there are symptoms, as well, full investigation should be carried out.

One further thought. Sudden, unexplained attacks of unconciousness in an apparently fit young person may be the first indication of a HOCM. Such patients are usually referred to the neurologist for an EEG. All should also have an echocardiogram.

If a HOCM is found, all but gentle exercise must be given up.

100. A GP goes to work as a clinical assistant to the local cardiologist. People often ask him the prognosis of their own, or their loved one's illness. Are there any areas of risk that could be much higher than the doctor might realise and which should be treated with healthy caution, rather than giving a cheerful grin and saying, 'Don't worry about that. He'll go on for years!'? And might a contrary situation exist where too much pessimism may be exercised?

In some specialities, such as oncology, prognosis is all-important and there are very many studies and hard statistics which will give the doctor a guide. They will not always turn out to be correct, but usually so. You can say, for example, that the vast majority of people with a carcinoma of the stomach with liver secondaries will be dead within twelve months. Few such hard and fast examples exist in cardiology.

I would suggest, therefore, that every doctor encountering patients with heart disease should have a little book, or a list, of some of the risks involved in cardiological medicine. Such a list would be too large to be included here. There are a number of surprises, many of which have already been discussed in this publication and its sister book *What Shall I Do? Questions and Answers in Cardiology*.

The death rate from heart attack, for example, in patients with chronic stable angina is only 2% per annum! On the other hand, unlike cancer, many sudden cardiological deaths occur in people who were assumed to be perfectly healthy and whose demise could not have been foreseen.

Elderly patients with CCF can go on for many years. There is a high rate of survival, and a surprisingly prolonged survival time, in patients who have had heart transplants. This must be borne in mind when considering a 50% mortality in 10 years for the teenager with HOCM, whereas in people who are older the 10-year mortality drops to 20%. In cardiomyopathy generally, echocardiography has enabled prognosis to be assessed much more accurately.

Ventricular ectopics are extremely common and constitute virtually no risk. There is hardly any risk of embolism from lone fibrillation – an entirely different situation exists in the patient with fibrillation and associated heart disease.

There is only a very small risk of death associated with cardiac catherisation, but there is a sufficient risk of other complications to justify it only being done in a unit with an attached cardiovascular surgical unit. The same applies, even more so, to angioplasty. CABG in cases of main stem disease and triple vessel disease increase life expectancy. As yet, angioplasty is of value for symptoms only. It has not been shown to improve survival.

A particular area of bad prognosis, if nothing is done, is aortic stenosis. Once the patient starts to faint or gets increasing angina, death is not far away.

Careful attention to patients with prosthetic heart valves is justified by the 50% mortality produced by SBE in such people, however fit and otherwise well they may be. This compares, paradoxically, with the habituated i/v drug addict whose SBE only carries about a 10% mortality – because it is usually right-sided.

The relative value of drugs and their effect on prognosis has to be known. Streptokinase and aspirin, ACE inhibitor and beta-blocker, all have their place to play in increasing survival time. The figures should be known when placing the options of treatment before the patient.

Index

Note: The numbers in this index refer to questions and not to pages.

Hysterectomy and Vaginal Repair, Sally Haslett, RGN, RHV, RM and Molly Jennings MCSP, 28pp, 3rd edn 1992, ISBN 0906584310

Explains the meaning and effect of these operations and describes how to prepare for them. Advice on what to do afterwards for a trouble-free return to normal life.

> *'This booklet has proved its worth over and over again.'*
>
> Woman's Realm

Having Gynaecological Surgery, Sally Haslett, RGN, RHV, RM and Molly Jennings MCSP, 30pp, 1995, ISBN 0986584396

Parallel booklet with the above, with advice on preparation for and recovery from gynaecological surgery other than hysterectomy or vaginal repair.

Having a Cervical Smear, Sally Haslett, RGN, RHV, RM, 21pp, 1994, ISBN 0906584388

Answers questions by women. Describes the test, the different investigations and treatments, and explains the technical terms that a doctor or nurse might use.

Lymphoedema: Advice on Treatment, Dr Claud Regnard, Caroline Badger RGN and Dr Peter Mortimer, 24pp, 2nd edn 1991, ISBN 0906584329

Explains what the condition is, and provides a daily management plan that can be followed at home.

> *'This little booklet is a model of a guide to self-help.'* Patient Voice

Oral Morphine: Information for Patients, Families and Friends, Dr Robert Twycross and Dr Sylvia Lack, 24pp, 1988, ISBN 0906584221

Brings together answers to questions frequently asked by patients.

> *'Answers many of the questions raised by patients and families when morphine is introduced in the treatment of cancer pain.'*
>
> Palliative Medicine

The Early Days of Grieving, Revd Derek Nuttall, 26pp, 1991, ISBN 0906584299

Offers support, explanation and information, speaking directly to the bereaved person.

> *'The author does this without becoming sentimental, mawkish or doctrinaire.'* The Lancet